The Productivity of Health Care and Pharmaceuticals

D1524316

The Productivity of Health Care and Pharmaceuticals

An International Comparison

H. E. Frech III
and
Richard D. Miller Jr.

The AEI Press

Publisher for the American Enterprise Institute
WASHINGTON, D.C.

1999

Available in the United States from the AEI Press, c/o Publisher Resources Inc., 1224 Heil Quaker Blvd., P.O. Box 7001, La Vergne, TN 37086-7001. Distributed outside the United States by arrangement with Eurospan, 3 Henrietta Street, London WC2E 8LU England.

Library of Congress Cataloging-in-Publication Data

Frech, H. E.
    The productivity of health care and pharmaceuticals : an international comparison / H. E. Frech, III, and Richard D. Miller, Jr.
        p.   cm.
    Includes bibliographical references and index.
    ISBN 0-8447-7124-4 (pbk. : alk. paper)
    1. Health   status   indicators—Research—Statistical methods.   2. Health status indicators—Statistics.
    3. Drug utilization—Research—Statistical methods.
    4. Drug utilization—Statistics.
I. Miller, Richard D., Jr.   II. Title.
RA407.F74   1999
362.1'04—dc21   98-48714
                                                       CIP

1 3 5 7 9 10 8 6 4 2

THE AEI PRESS
Publisher for the American Enterprise Institute
1150 17th Street, N.W., Washington, D.C. 20036

Printed in the United States of America

Contents

Preface

Background. Much work has analyzed the determinants of health care expenditures. Much less effort has centered on the determinants of health itself. This analysis focuses on the production of health, with special attention paid to disaggregating health care into pharmaceuticals and other health care. We also analyze the effects of wealth and certain lifestyles on health.

Researchers who have analyzed the determinants of health across geographic units have found certain striking and consistent results. First, basic public health services, in the form of potable water and sanitation services, provide the biggest payoffs in decreased mortality for all age groups, whereas the expansion of health care services does not improve mortality as much, if at all. Second, in studies that have analyzed developing countries, researchers have found that higher incomes are negatively related to mortality, while other researchers have found exactly the opposite result when they have limited their samples to rich countries or regions of those countries. Lifestyle factors have also been important determinants of health in many studies. Finally, the few studies that have examined the effect of pharmaceutical consumption on health outcomes in an international comparison context have been seriously flawed.

Methods. This study represents an improvement over these previous ones. We analyze a sample of twenty-one member-countries of the Organization for Economic Cooperation and Development (OECD) as of the early 1990s. Pharmaceutical and total health care expenditures are converted to U.S. dollars by using exchange rates for purchasing power parity for pharmaceuticals and health care, respectively. The OECD provided the purchasing power parities. The measures of pharmaceutical and other health care consumption used here are the best available for a *large* number of OECD countries. We measure each country's health crudely but objectively, with life expectancies at birth, at age forty, and at age sixty, along with infant mortality.

We use multivariate regressions to estimate production functions for health. The functional form allows for diminishing returns in each input in the production functions. The explanatory variables in each regression include pharmaceutical consumption, other health care consumption, gross domestic product, alcohol consumption, cigarette consumption, and richness of diet.

Findings. Our major finding is that pharmaceutical consumption has a positive and significant (both statistically and economically) effect on remaining life expectancy at age forty and at age sixty. It also has a smaller (although still positive) and statistically insignificant effect on life expectancy at birth. The elasticities of pharmaceutical consumption on life expectancy are roughly 0.017 at age forty and 0.040 at age sixty. The estimates are not sensitive to small changes in the analysis, such as restricting the sample to just the European countries. Expressed in terms of dollars per life year saved, the results indicate a large difference between high-use and low-use countries. For men aged forty, for example, our estimates range from more than $60,000 per life year saved in France to roughly $3,800 in Turkey. This difference is driven partially by the data and partially by the functional form used. Pharmaceutical consumption appears to have no significant effect on infant mortality, and, unfortunately, the infant mortality model is sensitive to small changes.

Nonpharmaceutical health care consumption appears to have no measurable effect on life expectancy, either at birth, at age forty, or at age sixty. Again, where infant mortality is concerned, the results are mixed and sensitive to small changes in the analysis. The gross domestic product has a positive and significant effect on life expectancies at the ages of forty and sixty, although this effect disappears in the European-only sample. The results from the infant mortality regressions are mixed.

The lifestyle variable with the biggest effect on health is dietary richness, measured by the consumption of animal fat. Increased richness of diet improves mortality up to a point, but the impact becomes negative as a diet becomes too rich. This result is somewhat surprising. One might have thought that the OECD countries are wealthy enough that nutrition, in this basic sense, would not be an issue.

This study should add to the debate over how OECD governments should allocate resources both among different health care goods and services and between health care and other goods and services. It improves on the existing literature because it uses better measures of pharmaceutical and other health care consumption and uses a functional form that allows for diminishing returns. The results have been surprising and robust in the life expectancy models. Increased pharmaceutical consumption helps improve mortality outcomes, especially for those at middle age and beyond.

Acknowledgment

The authors are grateful to the Chair in the Economics and Management of Health, Institut d'Etudes Politiques (Sciences Po) de Paris, for financial support. We also wish to thank Patricia Danzon, Jean-Jacques Rosa, Nathalie Vande Maele, David Roberts, Jean-Pierre Poullier, Manfred Huber, and J. Michael Woolley for helpful comments. Earlier versions of this monograph were presented at the University of California, Los Angeles; the University of California, Berkeley; the Ad Hoc Group on Pharmaceutical Economics in New York; and Interpharma in Basel, Switzerland. We are grateful to the participants in those seminars, especially William Comanor, Thomas Rice, Thomas Cueni, Richard Scheffler, Ted Keeler, Richard Manning, Allison Keith, and Peter Zweifel.

1
Introduction

There have been many international studies of health care, especially in the member-countries of the Organization for Economic Cooperation and Development (OECD). Mostly driven by budgetary and cost-containment problems, the vast majority have focused on the determinants of health care expenditures. The researchers have found that income, usually measured as gross domestic product, is a major determinant of health expenditures, with richer countries spending far more than poorer countries. Many have found results consistent with an income elasticity of greater than one, indicating that health care may be a luxury good even in rich countries.[1] The impact of economic institutions and policies on health expenditures has been mixed.

The emphasis on estimating the effects of different factors on health care spending is not entirely misplaced, but more effort should be devoted to estimating the determinants of health. Such estimates can help guide policymakers in how to allocate resources most effectively both among different types of health care goods and services and between health care and other goods. A few researchers from a variety of fields, including economics, epidemiology, sociology, and anthropology, have considered the effects of different factors on the production of health. The results of these studies have been mixed, and many of them have been flawed. Chapter 2 details this literature.

The particular focus of this research is the production of health, with special attention to disaggregating health care into pharmaceutical and other health care.

We focus on the productivity of pharmaceuticals in particular because pharmaceutical consumption varies considerably, even among the rich countries of Europe, North America, and Oceania. In 1990, for instance, France's per capita consumption of pharmaceuticals was five times that of Denmark, and Italy's was roughly twice that of the United States. A common belief holds that, among rich countries, the marginal return to health care consumption in general and pharmaceutical consumption in particular is negligible. Taken together, this leads to the belief that many rich countries, such as France and Italy, consume too many pharmaceuticals (*New York Times* 1991; *Washington Post* 1988). The popular press has accused doctors in countries such as Japan of overprescribing drugs (*Economist* 1996). Are those societies that consume more pharmaceuticals acting irrationally, or is there a measurable health return to such consumption?

To attempt to answer this question, a sample of twenty-one OECD countries as of the early 1990s is analyzed. Measuring pharmaceutical consumption is surprisingly tricky, but the measure of pharmaceutical consumption used here is the best one available for a large number of OECD countries. Each country's health is measured crudely but objectively, with life expectancies at various ages (birth, age forty, and age sixty), along with infant mortality. Chapter 3 discusses the data and methodological issues concerning measurement of variables of interest.

The analysis consists of various multivariate regressions. By analogy to other production processes, the productivity of health should exhibit diminishing returns in each of its inputs. A functional form used in the regression analysis allows for this. The explanatory variables in each regression include pharmaceutical consumption, gross domestic product, other health care consumption, and three lifestyle variables: alcohol consumption, cigarette consumption, and richness of diet. The results indicate that pharmaceutical consumption is statistically significantly positively related with increased life expectancy at the ages of forty and sixty, even when the above factors are controlled for. The elasticities of pharmaceutical consumption for life expectancies at these ages are 0.017 and 0.040, respectively. Doubling pharmaceutical consumption would raise life expectancy by about one year for those already sixty. If the analysis is limited to Europe, the positive effect is even larger. The results also indicate that richness of diet is important but that returns to enriching a country's diet can become negative. A more detailed description of the analyses follows in chapter 4.

2

A Review of the Literature

A number of studies bear on the productivity of medical care in improving health, and a few focus particularly on the productivity of drugs themselves. The quality, purpose, and approach of the studies vary greatly. Our review focuses on studies that relate most closely to our own work.

Aggregate Studies of the Production of Health

Areas within the United States. In an important early study of the production of health using cross-sectional data from the United States, Richard Auster, Irving Leveson, and Deborah Sarachek (1969) considered the relationship between mortality and both medical care and environmental variables.[1] They used a regression analysis of state aggregates for 1960. Medical care was measured in two ways: first, by total per capita medical care expenditures and second, by the output of a Cobb-Douglas production function, combining the services of physicians, other medical personnel, capital, and drugs. The environmental variables included per capita income, education levels, percentage of population in urban areas, percentage employed in manufacturing, alcohol consumption per capita, percentage in white-collar occupations, percentage of females not in the labor force, and the presence of a medical school in the state. The authors presented results from both an ordinary least squares regression and from two-stage least squares models where medical spending was treated as endogenous.

The key result of this study is that the environmental variables are much more important in determining the age-adjusted death rate than medical care is. The authors found education to be negatively associated with mortality rates in all regressions, while per capita income is positively associated with mortality rates. The latter result may have been due to the unfavorable diet, the sedentary and generally unhealthy lifestyle, and the greater psychological stress presumably associated with higher income. This negative partial effect of income on health is sometimes called the fast-lane lifestyle effect. The authors claimed that this could explain the poor U.S. performance in reducing mortality. Neither of the medical care measures significantly affected the age-adjusted death rate in the two-stage models.

In two studies, Jack Hadley (1982, 1988) estimated a series of health production functions using aggregate, U.S. cross-sectional data for 1970 and 1980. In the first study, he used the county group as the geographic unit of analysis[2] and focused on age-sex-race–specific mortality rates for eight adult and four infant population cohorts. Data came from the 1970 census and from special mortality files created under the sponsorship of the National Center for Health Statistics. Three approaches to defining medical care use were investigated: (1) the ratios of physicians, nurses, and acute care hospital beds per 1,000 people in the county group; (2) cohort-specific estimates of these ratios; and (3) Medicare expenditures per Medicare enrollee in the county group. Hadley found the third measure to be the best on both theoretical and empirical grounds. He estimated that, except for middle-aged males, a 10 percent increase in per capita medical care use is associated with about a 1.5 percent decrease in mortality rates. He also found that education is negatively related to mortality rates. For infants, he found that a 10 percent increase in total family income lowers infant mortality by 1.6–2.2 percent (except for black male infants); the effect of total family income on adult mortality is more ambiguous.

Hadley (1988) replicated his earlier study by using 1980 data and focusing on the elderly. He used the redefined county group as the geographic unit of analysis.[3] For whites, he found that a 10 percent higher level of Medicare spending per beneficiary is associated with mortality rates that range from 2.53 to 4.40 percent lower, depending on age and sex. The impact on African-American mortality is even greater, usually at least twice as great as for whites. The age cohort that experiences the greatest impact is the seventy- to seventy-four-year-old age group, regardless of race or sex. Not surprisingly, he also found that higher Medicare spending has the least impact on deaths from external causes, such as accidents and murder.

International Studies. Charles Stewart (1971) conducted an early analysis of international data to determine the productivity of health care. He divided the resources devoted to health into four categories: treatment, prevention, information, and research. Life expectancy was used as a dependent variable and was regressed on treatment variables (such as numbers of medical personnel and numbers of hospital beds), literacy rates (a proxy for information), and the availability of potable water (a proxy for prevention). The study was a cross-sectional analysis considering all nations in the Western Hemisphere as of the mid-1960s. Stewart found both literacy and the availability of potable water to be significantly related to life expectancy but found that none of the treatment variables mattered. Stewart noted that mortality rates are typically understated and that the extent of the understatement is greatest in the least-developed countries. Also, literacy rate differences are probably understated in the data because literacy standards tend to be lower in those countries with lower literacy rates.

Despite these misgivings about the data, Stewart comes to two general conclusions about the United States and its less-developed neighbors. First, the United States seems to be on the flat of the curve for the productivity of health care. In other words, the marginal effect on mortality of any resource devoted to prevention, information, or treatment is small in the United States. The best bet may be to increase research and development to improve the productivity of resources devoted to treatment. In the less-developed countries of the Western Hemisphere, all health resources should be devoted to prevention. More sanitary engineers and fewer doctors should be trained in these countries. This view is consistent with historical experience (Fuchs 1974, 31–53).

A. L. Cochrane, A. S. St. Leger, and F. Moore (1978) studied the relationship between various health service inputs and various mortality measures by using a cross-section of eighteen developed countries as of 1970. They limited their sample to those countries in which per capita gross national product was at least roughly $2,000 in 1970 and where the population exceeded 2 million. They also excluded Japan since they were concerned that genetic factors may account for a substantial proportion of any difference in mortality between it and the other, mostly European, countries that constituted the final sample. They used both simple correlations and regression analyses. In the regression analyses, they regressed maternal, infant, and perinatal mortality, along with mortality rates for various age groups, on the number of doctors, per capita GNP, cigarette consumption, alcohol consumption, population density, percentage of health care provided by public funds, and sugar consumption.

In general, the results of the study are mixed. First, the researchers found that a greater number of doctors is related to higher mortality rates in most age groups and for mothers and infants. This is true even of pediatricians and their effect on infant, perinatal, and maternal mortality. They also found per capita GNP negatively correlated with all mortality measures. Cigarette consumption appears to be positively correlated with all types of mortality,

7

though significant only in the regressions for infant and perinatal mortality. The results for alcohol consumption are more mixed, with a positive effect on infant mortality (significant) and maternal mortality (insignificant) but a negative, albeit insignificant, effect on mortality for those older than thirty-five. Finally, the percentage of health care provided through public funds has a negative, though statistically insignificant, effect on mortality, except for those between the ages of fifteen and thirty-five, where the effect is significant.

Many studies have found per capita income a powerful variable in explaining various measures of a society's health level. G. B. Rodgers (1979) included a measure of income inequality, the Gini coefficient, to determine its effect on life expectancy at birth, life expectancy at the fifth birthday, and infant mortality across countries. It makes sense that income inequality would influence health, holding average income constant, because of strongly diminishing returns to the income-health relationship. In his sample of fifty-six countries, Rodgers found that greater income inequality is associated with lower life expectancies both at birth and at the age of five and is associated with higher infant mortality rates. In his regressions, he included only per capita income and the Gini coefficient. Still, his analysis has the advantage of accounting for the decreasing returns of economic development, as measured by income per capita, in the production of health. Rodgers tried different functional forms, and his results are fairly robust. His basic result is that the difference in life expectancy between a fairly egalitarian society and a relatively nonegalitarian society is likely to be as much as five to ten years. It would be interesting to see if this result were robust to the inclusion of variables for environmental and health care spending.

Barbara Wolfe (1986) and Barbara Wolfe and Mary Gabay (1987) explored the hypothesis that lifestyle changes must be included to capture the true relationship between medical expenditures and health status in international comparisons. They considered twenty-two developed countries over twenty years. In the second paper, a simultaneous equation model is used. Changes in lifestyle, aging of the population, and changes in occupational risk were modeled as influences on medical expenditures. In the second stage, changes in medical expenditures and changes in lifestyle were modeled as determinants of the change in health status. The authors found a positive relationship between changes in real medical care expenditures and changes in life expectancy (although these relationships are not statistically significant at the usual levels).

The lack of statistical significance could be due to an overtaxing of the data. A two-stage estimation in first differences was probably too much for such a small data set to bear. First differencing alone may result in mostly noise; see Anand and Ravallion (1996). Further, two-stage least squares behaves badly when the first stage fits poorly (Nelson and Startz 1990). Although the first stage was not reported, we suspect that it does fit poorly.

In the study most similar to ours in its focus on OECD countries, Peter Zweifel and Matteo Ferrari (1992) considered what they call the Sisyphus syndrome in health care: increased medical care expenditures tend to prolong life, especially at advanced ages, and there is a positive feedback in that more consumers at advanced ages then drive up demand for health care and drive up expenditures. From a cost-containment perspective, the developed countries may be victims of their own medical care successes. Zweifel and Ferrari attempted to find evidence of this syndrome in aggregate data from the OECD countries.

The result of most interest to us concerns the first link in the Sisyphus syndrome. Zweifel and Ferrari found a positive relationship between total health care expenditures and life expectancy beyond the age of forty even when controlling for per capita gross domestic product, a result similar to Hadley's (1988). They found this result in

9

a regression where they lagged both health care expenditures and per capita gross domestic product by ten years. Another interesting result supporting the idea of the fast-lane lifestyle is the finding that lagged gross domestic product has a negative and significant effect on life expectancy, echoing Auster, Leveson, and Sarachek (1969).

In an attempt to estimate the positive feedback relationship, Zweifel and Ferrari found that remaining life expectancies beyond forty are not statistically significantly related to health care expenditures regardless of the specification or estimation method chosen. They concluded that the Sisyphus syndrome does not exert enough force to be detected in these data.

Sudhir Anand and Martin Ravallion (1993) examined the nature of the relationship between per capita real income and two measures of human development that we also consider: life expectancy and infant mortality. Their sample consisted of a cross-section of twenty-two poorer, developing countries as of the mid-1980s. Three possible explanations are presented for the commonly found relationship between per capita income and health. First, the capability to produce health is expanded directly through economic growth. Second, this capability is expanded through the reduction of poverty.[4] Finally, the capability to produce health is expanded through expanded social services, particularly medical services.

To determine which of these explanations is most powerful, Anand and Ravallion first regressed life expectancy on per capita income alone and found a strong and positive correlation between these two variables. They then added the proportion of the population consuming less than $1 per day in 1985—to control for poverty—and a measure of public health spending per person. When they did this, the correlation between life expectancy and per capita income disappeared, while the coefficient on per capita public health spending was positive and significant and the coefficient on the poverty measure was negative and significant. They concluded that average affluence matters to the extent that it leads to a lower poverty level and pays for better public health services. They then explained the impressive record of Sri Lanka in its progress in measured health, despite being a poor country, as a result of its high public health expenditures.

Howard Wall (1996) argued that Anand and Ravallion's results likely stemmed from their lack of control for fixed effects—such as diet, culture, and location—that are correlated with their regressors. Wall ran similar regressions with panel data from two years in the early 1980s on twenty-five developing countries, with country dummy variables to control for the fixed effects. He found that differences in per capita public health expenditure do not affect the positive relationship between per capita income and life expectancy. At the same time, he found that per capita income has a much less significant effect on life expectancy in the fixed-effects regression including only per capita income and a year dummy.

This tenuous effect of income on life expectancy leads Anand and Ravallion (1996) to reply that Wall's result is most likely due to measurement error bias, which tends to be more problematic in fixed-effects models. Measurement error in the regressors in fixed-effects models tends to bias coefficient estimates toward zero, which can explain the lack of explanatory power in per capita income in Wall's regression. It can also explain the lack of explanatory power of per capita public health spending, a variable likely to be measured with more error than per capita income.

Still, Anand and Ravallion's analysis could be improved. First, they put much emphasis on *public* health expenditure per capita, but they never investigated whether their measure of public health expenditure was acting merely as a proxy for total (public plus private) health expenditure. Also, data available on nutritional factors—see Gage and O'Connor (1994)—could be included. In general, public health expenditures should have an impact in poorer countries since the public sector provides those health services (sanitation, clean water, etc.) that have the biggest impact on health in poorer countries, but making the above improvements would make their argument stronger.

Sam Peltzman (1987) found similar effects of income distribution in a study that focused on the effects of pharmaceutical prescriptions. He chose twenty-two middle-income countries with per capita incomes between 5 percent and 50 percent of the U.S. level. He examined the death rate from poisoning and from infectious diseases for people between the ages of twenty and sixty-four. The interesting results follow.

First, median income is negatively related to mortality, but, with the median constant, a higher mean income (greater income inequality) implies higher mortality. This result is quite similar to Rodgers's (1979) and Anand and Ravallion's (1993), though different measures of income inequality were used. Second, the only significant effect of pharmaceutical regulation is a strong positive relationship between such regulation and the death rate from poisoning. Perhaps this results from forcing consumers to use black market drugs, or perhaps it results from reverse causation. Mandatory prescription requirements also appear to have a positive effect on the demand for doctors, and for some illnesses this indirect effect appears to improve health. Peltzman found no direct effect of regulation on the degree to which consumers realize benefits from pharmaceutical utilization.

Finally, a broad measure of government intervention, government health expenditures per dollar of GNP, appears, if anything, negatively related with life expectancy. Peltzman pointed out the sharp contrast between the effect of regulation and government intervention (bad) and the effect of diffuse economic development (good). This is exactly the opposite of the results and interpretation of Anand and Ravallion (1993), who argued that economic development leads to better health through increased spending on public health services.

Peltzman did study more developed countries, where the productive public investments in sanitation and clean water are more or less complete.

In another recent study, Martin Baily and Alan Garber (1998) investigated the productivity of the health care sectors in the United States, the United Kingdom, and Germany. Specifically, they looked at the treatment in each country of the following four diseases: diabetes, cholelithiasis (gallstones), breast cancer, and lung cancer. Inputs into the treatment of these diseases included labor inputs from physicians, nurses, and other providers; supplies such as medications, surgical instruments, and X-ray film; and physical capital such as diagnostic equipment and hospitals. They measured outcomes as either increases in life years (for breast and lung cancer) or increases in quality-adjusted life years (for cholelithiasis and diabetes).

Germany apparently devoted the most medical care resources to the treatment of each disease whereas the United Kingdom devoted the least. Still, Baily and Garber found no clear generalizable relationship between the level of medical resources used and outcomes. Germany, for instance, used 38 percent and 21 percent more resources than the United States in the treatment of breast and lung cancer, respectively. At the same time, Germany experienced outcomes that were only roughly 90 percent as favorable as the outcomes experienced in the United States for these two diseases. Conversely, in the case of cholelithiasis, Germany devoted 72 percent more resources to treatment than the United States, with outcomes that were 10 percent better than in the United States. Despite devoting 50 percent more resources to the treatment of diabetes, the United States experienced outcomes inferior to those in the United Kingdom. No clear trend indicates that the higher use of medical resources leads to better health outcomes.

Still, the findings should be taken only as suggestive. First, Baily and Garber failed to control for lifestyle differences across the countries. Second, they did not disaggregate the resources used into their components to determine which components were productive and which were unproductive. Was Germany's lack of productivity, for instance, due to unnecessarily long hospital stays or possibly due to the overprescription of pharmaceuticals? Finally, the study considered only four conditions in only three countries. Still, the investigation is useful in shedding light on the differences in treatment patterns across what most researchers would think are fairly homogeneous technologically advanced countries.

Political scientists Edmund Wnuk-Lipinski and Raymond Illsley (1990) examined health and inequality in the former Eastern bloc countries of Bulgaria, Hungary, Poland, and the Soviet Union. In simple cross-correlation and regression analyses, they found evidence that dysfunctions of these health systems are only minor contributing factors in the poor performance in these countries in mortality and life expectancy. The more fundamental causes of this poor performance are cultural and collective behavior and the priorities of the political and economic systems. Again, this is evidence of the importance of lifestyle and environmental factors in yet another set of countries.

Other noneconomists working in this field, Hugh Lena and Bruce London (1993), investigated the impact of selected political and economic processes on the well-being of populations within samples of fifty to eighty-four peripheral and noncore (sociological terms for developing) nations. More specifically, the authors studied the impact of specific factors—regime ideology, state strength (as measured by government expenditures as a proportion of GNP), multinational corporate penetration, and position in the world economy—on infant mortality, child death rate, and life expectancy. Even when controlling for per capita gross national product, the authors found that political systems matter in determining health and well-being. High levels of democracy and strong left-wing regimes are associated with positive health outcomes, and strong right-wing regimes are associated with lower life expectancies and higher mortality levels. This result could be a proxy for more egalitarian income distributions; if so, the results are consistent with Rodgers's (1979), Anand and Ravallion's (1993), and Peltzman's (1987).

Erica Hertz, James Herbert, and Joan Landon (1994) used data from United Nations sources for an international comparison of infant and maternal mortality rates and life expectancy at birth. Their sample consisted of a cross-section of sixty-six countries at all levels of economic development. Given that the sample included both developing and rich countries, not surprisingly they found that availability of sanitation facilities shows the strongest association with all three dependent variables, lowering both infant and maternal mortality and raising life expectancy. They also found the total literacy rate, total calorie consumption, and dietary composition to be important determinants of health. Variables for the availability of medical care resources, such as the availability of medical care personnel and the number of hospital beds per capita, do not significantly affect any dependent variables. These results are quite similar to those found by earlier researchers, such as Stewart (1971) and Auster and colleagues (1969) in the economics literature. A major flaw with the study is the use of stepwise regression techniques, which undermines statistical inference and interpretation; see Greene (1993).

Timothy Gage and Kathleen O'Connor (1994) examined the associations between nutrition and mortality at the national level. Their sample included both developing and rich countries. The results indicate that life expectancy is positively related to total calories, the total quality and quantity of diet, and the ratio of fats to protein. The ratio of carbohydrates to fats is positively associated with life expectancy. Higher ratios of fats to proteins are healthy initially, but the effect reverses when diets are rich. All effects of nutrition diminish considerably at high nutrient availability. This does not surprise an economist since it indicates that increased diet quality exhibits diminishing returns in the production of health.

This finding also reflects the epidemiological transition, the shift from infectious to degenerative causes of mortality. As a population's wealth increases, more resources can be made available for sanitation and clean water, and diets can become richer. At lower income levels, richer diets decrease mortality from infectious pathogens such as parasites and bacteria. At higher income levels, diets may become too rich and then lead to an increase in the number of cases of heart disease, cancer, and strokes, the leading causes of mortality in richer countries. Degenerative diseases are more likely to strike at advanced ages; the epidemiological transition is partially a byproduct of the success in fighting off infectious diseases and thus living to advanced ages. A flaw in the study of Gage and O'Connor is that income and other environmental variables such as education levels and the availability of clean water and sanitation were not included. Therefore, the decrease in mortality attributed to nutritional factors may be at least partially due to these other factors. The study does indicate that nutrient availability may be important, at least for developing countries.

The Productivity of Drugs across Nations. Akira Babazono and Alan Hillman (1994) used OECD data to investigate the effects of different components of medical care expenditures on perinatal and infant mortality and on male and female life expectancy. This work is closely related to ours because it examined the effects of drug use. In a 1988 cross-section of twenty-one OECD countries, Babazono and Hillman found that per capita pharmaceutical expenditures have no effect on these basic health measures. They also found that total health care spending per capita and inpatient and outpatient utilization are not related to health outcomes. But the work has many substantial flaws. First, the researchers blindly used the OECD data "as is," without critical thought to the difficulties inherent in comparing measures of different variables across countries and health systems. The authors, for example, included a variable for average length of hospital stays in different countries without considering that hospitals serve quite different functions in different countries. Primitive convalescent homes are considered hospitals in Japan whereas in the United States they are not. The authors compared average lengths of stay in different types of institutions. Another flaw is the authors' arrival at their final results by using a stepwise regression analysis, which leads to misleading statistical inference.

Perhaps most serious, drug consumption was badly mismeasured in this study. The authors used per capita pharmaceutical expenditures, converted to U.S. dollars according to exchange rates of gross domestic product purchasing power parity. As shown in the next chapter, these economywide purchasing power parities provide inaccurate measures of relative drug prices.[5] The use of these purchasing power parities led to mismeasurement of real drug consumption. Finally, the functional form used in the analysis is flawed since it does not allow for diminishing marginal productivity of pharmaceutical consumption in the production of health.

Other Studies of the Productivity of Pharmaceuticals. Other researchers have looked at microlevel data to determine the productivity of pharmaceuticals. Frank Lichtenberg (1996) analyzed the effects of changes in the quantity and types of pharmaceuticals prescribed by doctors on rates of hospitalization, surgical procedures, and mortality. He obtained data on drugs prescribed by physicians from the 1980 and 1991 National Ambulatory Medical Care Survey (NAMCS) Drug Mentions files. To analyze the relationship between changes in the pattern of drug use and changes in other medical inputs and mortality, Lichtenberg computed disease-level aggregate statistics from six additional sources, including the NAMCS 1980

17

and 1991 patient files, the 1980 and 1992 National Hospital Discharge Survey files, and the 1980 and 1991 Vital Statistics–Mortality Detail files. He found that for those diseases involving the greatest increases in both quantity and novelty of pharmaceuticals, the number of hospital stays, bed-days, and surgical procedures declined most rapidly. Also, increases in pharmaceutical quantity and novelty are associated with reductions in the number of both hospital deaths and deaths per hospital stay. Nonhospital mortality is unaffected, as is the mean age of death.

In another recent study, David Cutler, Mark McClellan, and Joseph Newhouse (1997) considered the factors that have led to reduced mortality from cardiovascular disease. Part of their analysis consists of a comprehensive review of the literature that has addressed trends in advanced myocardial infarction patient characteristics, treatment outcomes, and the cost of care from the mid-1970s to the mid-1990s. The researchers found that, from 1984 to 1991, life expectancy after a heart attack rose by 8 percent. They reported that a substantial portion of this improvement in mortality was due to changes in treatment such as the use of aspirin, beta blockers, and thrombolytic drugs. To a lesser extent, certain invasive surgical procedures also helped. Conversely, changes in factors related to personal behavior played a far more limited role. In other words, the results of this study indicate that pharmaceutical consumption plays a much more important role in lower mortality rates for patients with cardiovascular disease than any other factor.

A number of studies have also investigated the effects of restricted formularies imposed on the Medicaid population by some U.S. states. In the U.S. Medicaid program, the federal government leaves the states free to select which prescription drugs to reimburse patients for and which drugs not to reimburse them for. Under restricted formularies, states limit the availability of pharmaceuticals to their Medicaid populations (Grabowski 1988). As of 1990, twenty states had such restricted formularies.

William Moore and Robert Newman (1993) used a multivariate regression model to analyze pooled cross-sectional state data for the years 1985–1989. They estimated the effect of restricted formularies on total Medicaid expenditures, Medicaid reimbursements for prescription drugs, and Medicaid reimbursements for other types of health care. The authors controlled for both state and various Medicaid program characteristics. The results indicate that the formularies decrease expenditures on prescription drugs (by 13 percent) but leave total Medicaid expenditures unchanged. This is due mostly to a 33 percent increase in mental patient hospital expenses and a 25 percent increase in physician services expenses. This result indicates that prescription drug consumption is productive in the Medicaid population and that without access to the drugs, Medicaid patients must go to other sources to preserve their health stock.

In two other studies, Stephen Soumerai and colleagues (1991 and 1994) considered the effects of formularies on the elderly and on patients with schizophrenia. In the first study, they analyzed thirty-six months of Medicaid claims data from New Hampshire, which had a three-drug limit per patient for eleven of those months, and from New Jersey, which had no restrictions. The study patients were older than sixty years of age. Survival and time-series analyses were conducted to determine the effect of the restrictions in New Hampshire on admissions to hospitals and nursing homes. When the restrictions were instituted, drug use fell by 35 percent; this decrease was associated with an increase of admissions to nursing homes. No changes were observed in the New Jersey comparison group. When the restrictions were discontinued, the excess risk of nursing home admission ceased. This result is similar to Moore and Newman's and can be interpreted similarly.

In the second study, Soumerai and colleagues (1994) again investigated the effects of the restrictions in New Hampshire but focused on a population of schizophrenic patients. The study and comparison patients were permanently disabled, noninstitutionalized, and aged nineteen to sixty years of age. The restrictions resulted in reductions in the use of all psychotropic drugs (by 14–45 percent) and increases of one to two visits per patient per month to community mental health centers. Sharp increases in the use of emergency mental health services and partial hospitalization also occurred. After the restrictions were discontinued the use of medications and mental health services reverted to the previous level. Again, this is evidence that pharmaceuticals are important in producing health.

Summary

Where does this literature survey leave us? Certain results appear strong and make sense. First, basic public health services, in the form of a potable water supply and sanitation services, provide the biggest payoffs in decreased mortality for all age groups. These services are matters of civil engineering, not health care. This result has been found by all researchers who have studied underdeveloped countries and, in their work, have introduced a sufficient range in these public health infrastructure variables. Another striking and consistent result, the expansion of medical care services does not improve mortality rates nearly as much as public health infrastructure development does. As Stewart (1971) commented, the best thing for the less-developed countries to do would be to train more sanitation engineers and worry about training doctors only after the basic public health infrastructure was in place.

Environmental factors and per capita income have had a much greater effect on mortality than medical care. Higher levels of education are negatively related to mortality. Dietary factors have been found important, as richer diets tend to decrease mortality from infectious diseases, although at some point the rate of deaths from degenerative diseases begins to increase as diets become too rich. This is also true of income. At low income levels, increases in income tend to be associated with lower mortality rates. At higher income levels (in the most developed countries), income is positively related to mortality rates, at least when education is controlled for. Studies have also found that variation in alcohol and cigarette consumption can explain variation in mortality whereas variation in medical care utilization cannot. Finally, a few studies have suggested that the political environment may play a role in determining mortality.

While most studies have discovered little effect of more medical care on population mortality rates, the best-researched studies have found small negative effects. Hadley (1988) and Zweifel and Ferrari (1992) found such a relationship for older cohorts for areas within the United States and across countries. Hadley (1982) also reported such a relationship for younger cohorts in the United States, although he measured the health care consumption of older people.

Few studies, either directly or indirectly, have dealt with the effect of pharmaceutical consumption on mortality rates. Those studies dealing with this relationship directly have had serious flaws. In one of the better studies, Peltzman (1987) considered the effects of pharmaceutical regulations on national health indicators and found that mandatory prescription laws are positively related to mortality from poisonings. This relationship may reflect the perverse effects of the regulations, or it may reflect only reverse causation. The poisonings may have been the reason why such regulations were enacted in the first place. The microstudy by Lichtenberg (1996) and many studies of restricted formularies in the United States have also provided evidence that pharmaceutical consumption has a positive impact on health. It is our goal to investigate whether this effect can be found in an international comparison study.

21

3

Data and Methodological Issues

The Data

The data analyzed here came from the Organization for Economic Cooperation and Development. The OECD data set includes data on health care outcomes such as life expectancy for both males and females, potential years of life lost attributable to various causes, and infant and perinatal mortality. Other premature mortality and morbidity measures are included but are not available for many countries or for long periods. This is true of many other data series as well.

The data set includes statistics on medical determinants of health such as the number of inpatient beds per 1,000 inhabitants, the number of physicians and other health care professionals, and the number of hospital admissions. Although the data set reports information on health insurance coverage provided by public agencies, it does not cover private health insurance. This exclusion renders the insurance data almost useless. Total and public expenditures on various health care inputs, including pharmaceuticals, are also available. To facilitate cross-national comparisons, various exchange rates are provided to convert these expenditure levels into U.S. dollars. For the years 1980, 1985, 1990, and 1993, separate purchasing power parity (PPP) exchange rates are provided for pharmaceuticals and medical services. This is true for almost all countries in 1990 and 1993 and for most countries for 1980 and 1985.

Measuring Pharmaceutical Consumption

How one converts a nation's per capita pharmaceutical expenditures to U.S. dollars for the purpose of cross-national comparisons is crucial. Babazono and Hillman (1994) used PPP exchange rates designed to convert the total gross domestic product to U.S. dollars. This approach is appropriate only if pharmaceutical prices differ across countries in the same way that prices differ in general. Researchers who have looked at this issue in depth, including Tadeusz Szuba (1986) and Patricia Danzon and Allison Percy (1995), have demonstrated that this is far from the truth. Drug price regulation remains a national prerogative in many countries, and trade barriers have traditionally been significant. Both price regulation and barriers vary widely.

Biased (in favor of domestic producers) price regulation, for instance, is practiced in France and Italy. In this situation, a manufacturer's price must be approved for a product to be reimbursed by social insurance programs. This method keeps pharmaceutical prices particularly low in France and in Italy. Spain also strictly regulates pharmaceutical prices. Other OECD countries, such as the United Kingdom and Germany, regulate pharmaceutical prices, albeit indirectly and typically much less stringently.[1] The United States and Denmark, at the other extreme, generally permit free pricing of pharmaceuticals, subject to market forces. For these reasons, one might expect the exchange rates for the gross domestic product PPP to be unsatisfactory for converting pharmaceutical expenditures to U.S. dollars for cross-national comparisons.

Luckily, PPP exchange rates designed specifically for converting pharmaceutical expenditures to U.S. dollars are available for 1980, 1985, 1990, and 1993. Table 3–1 presents measures of per capita pharmaceutical expenditures converted to U.S. dollars by using pharmaceutical PPP exchange rates and gross domestic product PPP exchange rates for 1990. Conversions using gross domestic

TABLE 3–1
COMPARING MEASURES OF REAL PHARMACEUTICAL
CONSUMPTION BY PHARMACEUTICAL PURCHASING POWER
PARITY AND GDP PURCHASING POWER PARITY EXCHANGE
RATES, 1990

Rank	Country	Pharmaceutical PPPs	GDP PPPs	Difference
1	France	560.927	256.278	304.649
2	Italy	448.200	242.235	205.965
3	Germany	374.138	311.483	62.655
4	Belgium	304.466	193.561	110.904
5	Spain	286.618	144.749	141.870
6	Portugal	247.092	153.211	93.881
7	United States	231.000	231.000	0.000
8	Sweden	225.859	119.700	106.159
9	Norway	216.341	125.180	91.161
10	Greece	216.032	95.128	120.904
11	Canada	215.650	190.769	24.881
12	Australia	196.386	117.266	79.120
13	New Zealand	194.828	140.373	54.455
14	Austria	191.940	154.345	37.595
15	Finland	190.663	121.630	69.033
16	Switzerland	190.476	145.455	45.021
17	United Kingdom	183.721	131.667	52.054
18	Netherlands	130.189	127.189	3.000
19	Ireland	120.690	101.449	19.241
20	Denmark	112.846	95.421	17.425
21	Turkey	62.115	34.869	27.246

SOURCE: OECD (1996) and the authors' calculations.

product PPP exchange rates invariably underestimate actual pharmaceutical expenditures outside the United States. Using the pharmaceutical PPP exchange rate, for instance, yields a value of $561 for France, whereas the value is only $256 if using the gross domestic product PPP exchange rate. A similar result is found for Italy. The biggest differences occur in those countries with the strictest price regulations, France and Italy; this differential indicates that the pharmaceutical PPPs make sense.

Danzon and Percy (1995) argue that even the pharmaceutical PPP exchange rates are flawed and provide more accurate Fisher price indexes for a handful of countries to convert pharmaceutical expenditures to U.S. dollars.[2] These price indexes are painstakingly calculated by using detailed proprietary data that are available only for a few countries. These relative price measures should be regarded as the gold standard, as they are undoubtedly the most accurate. But they are not available for any countries other than France, Italy, Germany, and the United Kingdom. Further, the detailed prices were converted from other currencies into dollars by using market exchange rates, rather than purchasing power parity exchange rates. This method seems to have had little effect on the rankings of consumption of various countries, but it does seem to have compressed measured consumption, relative to the United States.

One can convert pharmaceutical consumption in France, Italy, Germany, and the United Kingdom to U.S. dollars by using the pharmaceutical PPP and the gross domestic product PPP exchange rates for 1980, 1985, and 1990. Danzon and Percy measures are also available for these countries in these three years. Correlations among the three measures of pharmaceutical consumption for these years and countries were calculated. The correlation between the Danzon and Percy measure and the pharmaceutical purchasing power parity measure is fairly high, at 0.872. The other two correlation coefficients are both roughly 0.5. These correlations indicate that the consumption measure using the pharmaceutical purchasing power parity exchange rates compares well with the Danzon and Percy measure.

Szuba (1986) painstakingly assembled price ratios from detailed proprietary data, though with a slightly different approach. His price coefficients are excellent—when available. Szuba's price coefficients are applied to expenditure data after they have been converted to U.S. dollars by using conventional market exchange rates (like

Danzon and Percy). He found that in 1983 Italy had the lowest pharmaceutical prices and that the United States had the highest pharmaceutical prices among the six countries he studied (listed in table 3–2). We apply his price coefficients to 1985 expenditure estimates, which have been converted to U.S. dollars by using the market exchange rates.

TABLE 3–2
COMPARING MEASURES OF REAL PHARMACEUTICAL
EXPENDITURES FOR 1985 IN SIX COUNTRIES WITH VARIOUS
CONVERSIONS TO U.S. DOLLARS

Country	Exchange Rate	GDP Purchasing Power Parities	Pharma- ceutical Purchasing Power Parities	Danzon & Percy's Fisher Price Index	Szuba's Price Coeffi- cients
France	129.48	176.36	401.38	387.16	556.20
Italy	94.30	148.00	269.96	258.97	457.06
Germany	174.15	229.60	257.29	290.83	256.79
Switzerland	102.44	115.07	135.84	NA	147.81
United States	150.00	150.00	150.00	150.00	150.00
United Kingdom	66.67	94.55	119.85	103.44	126.01

CORRELATIONS AMONG THE VARIOUS PHARMACEUTICAL
CONSUMPTION MEASURES

Exchange rate	1.000	0.988	0.527	0.686	0.225
GDP PPP		1.000	0.574	0.728	0.313
Pharmaceutical PPP			1.000	0.979	0.924
Danzon & Percy				1.000	0.851
Szuba					1.000

NA = Not applicable.
SOURCE: OECD (1996); Danzon and Percy (1995); Szuba (1986); and the authors' calculations.

Table 3–2 compares measures of real pharmaceutical expenditures for 1985 with the following conversion factors: market exchange rates, gross domestic product purchasing power parities, pharmaceuticals purchasing power parities, Danzon and Percy's Fisher price indexes, and Szuba's price coefficients. Again, we find differences, but a general pattern emerges. France seems to outspend the other countries significantly, with Italy and Germany at the next tier, with expenditures significantly higher than those in the United States. Switzerland and the United Kingdom tend to consume fewer pharmaceuticals than the United States no matter which measure is used.

Table 3–2 also presents correlations among the different measures for 1985. The measure that we used in our study is highly correlated with both the Danzon and Percy measure and the Szuba measure for the countries for which all measures are available. The measures that use simple market exchange rates and gross domestic product purchasing power parity exchange rates are not highly correlated with the Danzon and Percy or Szuba measures. The analyses described above, along with conversations with officers at the OECD, lead us to believe that using the pharmaceutical PPP exchange rates is a significant step forward from earlier work that used the gross domestic product PPP exchange rates. Since we wish to study more than the five countries for which Danzon and Percy provide price indexes, the pharmaceutical PPP exchange rates provided by OECD, however imperfect, are the best conversion factors available.

Our measure of pharmaceutical consumption should still be viewed as only a reliable approximation. The measure cannot capture all of the more subtle differences in pharmaceutical use across countries. Two countries may spend approximately the same amount of money on pharmaceuticals but still exhibit different patterns of consumption. Livio Garattini and his colleagues (1994), for example, attempted to analyze the prices of the 100 best-selling pharmaceuticals in 1992 in Italy, Germany,

France, and the United Kingdom. Only eight products were common to all four best-seller lists. The researchers also found that the proportions of pharmaceuticals sold in three different therapeutic classes varied considerably across the four countries. Danzon and Percy and Szuba also reported this to be the case. Thus, the measure of pharmaceutical consumption used in this research is hardly uniform across countries.

Health Indicators

So far we have discussed problems in the measurement of our explanatory variable of greatest interest. Now we turn to the dependent variables. Many previous researchers have focused on mortality because it is widely considered the most reliable health indicator, especially among the industrialized countries that routinely report vital statistics (Office of Technology Assessment 1993).[3] Focusing on mortality rates for less-developed countries can be more problematic. As Murray (1987) points out, recent empirical information on mortality exists for only a handful of the developing countries. Many published estimates of mortality in most developing countries are based on old surveys updated over the years with *assumed* rates of improvement in mortality. The mechanistic updating of old data undermines the credibility of the research on the developing countries. This is not a problem with our analysis, since we have limited our study to industrialized members of the OECD, which all routinely publish vital statistics on a yearly basis.

Life expectancies at birth and at various advanced ages have been used as health indicators in many of the previous studies cited, and we use them also. Infant mortality rates are also used as a health indicator. The Office of Technology Assessment (1993) finds no serious problems with the data from industrialized countries on life expectancy. OTA does urge caution in using cause-specific mortality rates because of international differences in diagnostic techniques, the use of autopsies, and the training of medical personnel.

Even among the richest countries, caution is prudent in using infant mortality in international comparisons. Physicians in the United States, for example, are more likely to resuscitate extremely premature and low-birthweight infants, who later die. These are classified as live births in the United States and thus are included in calculations of infant mortality. Other countries are more likely to classify such births as fetal deaths. In some countries, infants may be classified as stillbirths if they die before their births are registered, sometimes as many as two days after birth. In Japan, this problem is exacerbated by the fact that many infant deaths are recorded as stillbirths because the latter are not recorded in Koseki, the Japanese family registration system (OTA 1993). We exclude Japan from our analysis because of this and other problems with Japanese health care data.

Measures of infant mortality and of female and male life expectancy for the twenty-one countries included in the study for the years 1980, 1985, 1990, and 1993 are presented in table 3–3. The data show that each country, carrying on long-term trends, experienced improvements in each health indicator throughout the 1980s and into the early 1990s. As of 1993, infant mortality ranged from a low of 4.4 deaths per 1,000 live births in Finland to a high of 52.6 deaths per 1,000 live births in Turkey. Though still high by OECD standards, Turkey's infant mortality rate in 1993 was a significant improvement over what it had been only thirteen years earlier (95.3 deaths per 1,000 live births in 1980). Greece, Portugal, and Spain also experienced significant improvements in infant mortality throughout the 1980s and into the early 1990s.

Female life expectancy at birth in 1993 was highest in France and Switzerland at 81.4 years. No fewer than nine of the countries included enjoyed female life expectancies over 80 years. Turkey ranked lowest in female life expectancy in 1993, as in earlier years, at 70 years. As for

TABLE 3–3
HEALTH INDICATOR MEASURES FOR SELECTED COUNTRIES,
1980, 1985, 1990, AND 1993

Country	1980	1985	1990	1993
United States				
Infant mortality	12.6	10.6	9.2	8.4
Female life expectancy	77.4	78.2	78.8	78.8
Male life expectancy	70.0	71.1	71.8	72.2
Australia				
Infant mortality	10.7	9.9	8.2	6.1
Female life expectancy	78.1	78.8	80.1	80.9
Male life expectancy	71.0	72.4	73.9	75.0
Austria				
Infant mortality	14.3	11.2	7.8	6.5
Female life expectancy	76.1	77.3	78.9	79.4
Male life expectancy	69.0	70.4	72.4	73.0
Belgium				
Infant mortality	12.1	9.8	8.0	8.0
Female life expectancy	76.8	77.7	79.1	79.8
Male life expectancy	70.0	70.9	72.4	73.0
Canada				
Infant mortality	10.4	8.0	6.8	6.8
Female life expectancy	79.1	79.7	80.4	81.2
Male life expectancy	71.9	73.0	73.8	74.9
Denmark				
Infant mortality	8.4	7.9	7.5	5.4
Female life expectancy	77.6	77.5	77.7	77.6
Male life expectancy	71.4	71.6	72.0	72.3
Finland				
Infant mortality	7.6	6.3	5.6	4.4
Female life expectancy	77.6	78.5	78.9	79.5
Male life expectancy	69.2	70.1	70.9	72.1
France				
Infant mortality	10.0	8.3	7.3	6.4
Female life expectancy	78.4	79.4	80.9	81.4
Male life expectancy	70.2	71.3	72.7	73.3

TABLE 3–3 (continued)				
Country	*1980*	*1985*	*1990*	*1993*
Germany				
Infant mortality	12.7	8.9	7.1	5.8
Female life expectancy	76.6	78.1	79.1	79.3
Male life expectancy	69.9	71.5	72.7	73.8
Greece				
Infant mortality	17.9	14.1	9.7	8.5
Female life expectancy	76.6	78.9	79.4	79.9
Male life expectancy	72.2	74.1	74.6	74.9
Ireland				
Infant mortality	11.1	8.9	8.2	5.9
Female life expectancy	75.0	76.4	77.5	78.2
Male life expectancy	69.5	70.8	72.0	72.7
Italy				
Infant mortality	14.6	10.5	8.2	7.3
Female life expectancy	77.4	78.6	80.0	80.9
Male life expectancy	70.6	72.0	73.5	74.5
Netherlands				
Infant mortality	8.6	8.0	7.1	6.3
Female life expectancy	79.2	79.7	80.1	80.0
Male life expectancy	72.4	73.1	73.8	74.0
New Zealand				
Infant mortality	12.9	10.8	8.4	7.3
Female life expectancy	76.3	77.3	78.3	78.9
Male life expectancy	70.1	71.0	72.4	73.1
Norway				
Infant mortality	8.1	8.5	7.0	5.1
Female life expectancy	79.2	79.4	79.8	80.2
Male life expectancy	72.3	72.6	73.4	74.2
Portugal				
Infant mortality	24.3	17.8	11.0	8.7
Female life expectancy	75.9	76.7	77.9	78.0
Male life expectancy	67.7	69.7	70.9	70.8

(*continued*)

TABLE 3–3 (continued)				
Country	1980	1985	1990	1993
Spain				
Infant mortality	12.3	8.9	7.6	6.8
Female life expectancy	78.6	79.7	80.4	80.9
Male life expectancy	72.5	73.3	73.4	73.3
Sweden				
Infant mortality	6.9	6.8	6.0	4.8
Female life expectancy	78.8	79.7	80.4	80.8
Male life expectancy	72.8	73.8	74.8	75.5
Switzerland				
Infant mortality	9.1	6.9	6.8	5.6
Female life expectancy	78.8	80.1	80.9	81.4
Male life expectancy	72.3	73.4	74.0	74.7
Turkey				
Infant mortality	95.3	75.3	59.3	52.6
Female life expectancy	64.3	65.4	68.4	70.0
Male life expectancy	58.2	60.7	64.1	65.4
United Kingdom				
Infant mortality	12.1	9.4	7.9	6.3
Female life expectancy	75.9	77.4	78.6	78.9
Male life expectancy	70.2	71.5	72.9	73.6

SOURCE: OECD (1996).

male life expectancy at birth, Sweden ranked first in 1993, with a life expectancy of 75.5 years. Once again, Turkey ranked last, with a male life expectancy of 65.4 years. To keep the Turkish experience in perspective, this showing is a vast improvement over the life expectancy of a male Turk in 1980, only 58.2 years.

4

The Analysis

Specification Issues

Our primary interest is the determinants of the health of a nation's citizens. One useful starting point is to consider an individual's health as being determined by a number of different factors through a household production function.[1] These factors include the consumption of goods that may have either positive or negative effects on an individual's health. The consumption of cigarettes, for example, has been found to lead to increases in mortality, or lower life expectancies, because of emphysema, lung cancer, and heart disease. Meanwhile, epidemiological studies (Gage and O'Connor 1994) have found nutritional variables to affect life expectancy. The studies cited in the literature review indicate that the consumption of nonmedical goods, so-called lifestyle choices, is an important determinant of the health of a population, especially for rich countries.

Some of the better previous studies have indicated that goods and services provided by the medical care sector also help to determine the health of a population. Pharmaceutical products fall into this general category along with other health care services. One would expect the consumption of such goods and services to augment a population's health. In a market-oriented economy, any services that did not augment health would not long be demanded. Even in more centralized economies, one would expect public choice mechanisms to favor productive health care over useless health care.

We can think of a nation's health as a function of pharmaceutical consumption, other health care consumption, wealth, and lifestyle and environmental factors. Specifically, we use the life expectancies of males and females at birth, at the age of forty, and at the age of sixty, as of the year 1993, as proxies for the health of a nation's population. Infant mortality is considered separately. These measures are discussed more fully in "Empirical Results for Life Expectancy."

We measure per capita pharmaceutical consumption by converting 1985 per capita pharmaceutical expenditures to 1990 U.S. dollars. The choice of conversion method is based on the discussion of the previous section. We take the expenditures in the national currency and then multiply by the nation's 1985 pharmaceutical purchasing power parity exchange rate. This gives us a measure of expenditures valued in U.S. prices. Then we inflate the resulting figure to 1990 U.S. dollars by multiplying by the ratio of the U.S. consumer price index for 1990–1985.

No exchange rate for pharmaceutical purchasing power parity is available for Switzerland in 1985, though it is available for 1990. Based on conversations with OECD officials and others, the pharmaceutical PPP for the United Kingdom is suspect for 1985. Thus, for these countries, we use a slightly different procedure. In the Swiss example, we convert Swiss pharmaceutical expenditures to 1990 U.S. dollars by first converting 1985 Swiss pharmaceutical expenditures (in Swiss francs) to 1990 Swiss francs and using the ratio of the Swiss index of consumer prices for 1990–1985. This gives us 1985 Swiss spending in 1990 Swiss francs. We then convert this figure to U.S. dollars by using the Swiss pharmaceutical purchasing power parity exchange rate for 1990. A similar approach is taken with the United Kingdom.

The measure of other health care consumption is likewise constructed by converting 1985 per capita health care expenditures to 1990 U.S. dollars. For this, we first apply the nation's 1985 exchange rate for *health care* purchasing power parity and then the U.S. consumer price index. From this figure, the measure of per capita pharmaceutical consumption is subtracted. For Switzerland, the approach taken is similar to the one described for pharmaceuticals because the Swiss health care purchasing power parity exchange rate for 1985 is unavailable.

Living standards and other lifestyle factors are also controlled for. First, we include each nation's 1985 per capita gross domestic product converted to 1990 U.S. dollars. For the conversion, we use each nation's 1985 gross domestic product purchasing power parity exchange rate and the U.S. consumer price index. We also control for cigarette smoking by including the percentages of females and males aged fifteen years or older who smoked as of 1983. Alcohol consumption is controlled for by including each nation's 1983 alcohol consumption in liters per capita per year. Finally, the richness of diet is controlled for by including a measure of animal fat consumed per capita per day. This measure is constructed by subtracting the average animal protein calories consumed per day from the average total animal calories consumed per day.

In our specification, the explanatory variables are lagged by roughly ten years, because lifestyle factors and medical care consumption have a cumulative rather than a contemporaneous effect on health. (The exact lag depends on data availability.) We follow Zweifel and Ferrari (1992) in this. As an example of a cumulative effect, smoking kills people not immediately, but rather over a period of years. A full model of this general idea would require several lags of each explanatory variable. Limitations of both data and sample size lead us to include only one lag. First, our sample studies only twenty-one countries. Adding a large number of lagged explanatory variables would lead to a huge decrease in precious degrees of freedom. Second, purchasing power parity conversions for total health care and pharmaceuticals are available only for 1980, 1985, and 1990. Thus, we would be able to include lagged terms only for 1980 or 1990. Given the persistence of the explanatory variables over time, this method would most likely lead to a multicollinearity problem. Including lags from the 1960s or the 1970s could be worthwhile, but the necessary data do not exist.

Finally, we use a double-log, or constant-elasticity, functional form for several reasons. First, a coefficient from a double-log regression is interpreted as an elasticity: the percentage change in the value of the dependent variable associated with a 1 percent change in the value of an explanatory variable. Second, we desire a model specified to allow for diminishing returns to all independent variables. In the double-log model, the elasticity is held constant, and the absolute value of the marginal effect of each explanatory variable is forced to fall at higher and higher values of the explanatory variable. The data to which one applies such a model determine the rate at which the absolute marginal effect decreases.[2]

Descriptive Statistics

Descriptive statistics presented in table 4–1 indicate much variation in both the dependent variables to be explained and in the regressors to do the explaining. Pharmaceutical consumption per capita, for example, varies by a factor of almost twenty, from $28.64 in Turkey to $490.68 in France. Gross domestic product per capita varies by a factor of five, from $4,080 in Turkey to $19,876.53 in the United States. Lifestyles also vary widely among the countries in our sample. For convenience in checking and critiquing our work, tables B–1, B–2, and B–3 in the appendix present the entire data set used for this study.

Tables 4–2 and 4–3 provide simple cross-correlations among the variables included in the life expectancy regressions. Some correlations are fairly surprising. First, higher aggregate alcohol consumption appears correlated with higher female life expectancy and lower infant mortality. This is probably because men consume a preponderance of alcohol and aggregate alcohol consumption is

TABLE 4–1
DESCRIPTIVE STATISTICS

Variable	Mean	Standard Deviation	Minimum	Maximum
Dependent variables				
MLE	73.09	2.37	64.10	75.50
ln(MLE)	4.29	0.03	4.16	4.32
MLE40	35.60	1.34	31.70	37.30
ln(MLE40)	3.57	0.04	3.46	3.62
MLE60	18.44	0.99	16.00	19.70
ln(MLE60)	2.91	0.06	2.77	2.98
FLE	79.26	2.73	68.40	81.40
ln(FLE)	4.37	0.04	4.22	4.40
FLE40	40.87	1.58	36.00	42.90
ln(FLE40)	3.71	0.04	3.58	3.76
FLE60	22.65	1.36	18.40	24.60
ln(FLE60)	3.12	0.06	2.91	3.20
INFMORT	9.91	10.83	5.60	59.30
Regressors				
PHPC	201.59	96.00	28.64	490.68
ln(PHPC)	5.19	0.56	3.35	6.20
GDPPC	13,968.87	3,988.46	4,080.08	19,876.53
ln(GDPPC)	9.49	0.37	8.31	9.90
HEPC	1,221.38	568.22	141.36	2,335.83
ln(HEPC)	6.95	0.67	4.95	7.76
FEMSMOKE	27.10	7.30	9.00	42.50
ln(FEMSMOKE)	3.26	0.33	2.20	3.75
MALESMOKE	43.56	9.09	31.80	62.80
ln(MALESMOKE)	3.75	0.20	3.46	4.14
ALCOHOL	10.51	4.31	1.20	19.10
ln(ALCOHOL)	2.21	0.65	0.18	2.95
ANFAT	1,026.43	292.46	252.00	1,324.00
ln(ANFAT)	6.87	0.40	5.53	7.19

(continued)

TABLE 4–1 (continued)

NOTE:

Variable	Definition
Dependent variables	
MLE	Male life expectancy at birth, 1993
MLE40	Male life expectancy at age 40, 1993
MLE60	Male life expectancy at age 60, 1993
FLE	Female life expectancy at birth, 1993
FLE40	Female life expectancy at age 40, 1993
FLE60	Female life expectancy at age 60, 1993
INFMORT	Infant mortality (deaths per 1,000 live births), 1990
Explanatory variables	
PHPC	Pharmaceutical expenditures per capita, 1985 (in 1990 U.S.$)
GDPPC	Gross domestic product per capita, 1985 (in 1990 U.S.$)
HEPC	Health expenditures (not including pharmaceuticals) per capita, 1985 (in 1990 U.S.$)
FEMSMOKE	Percentage of females aged 15 years or older who smoke, 1983
MALESMOKE	Percentage of males aged 15 years or older who smoke, 1983
ALCOHOL	Alcohol consumption in liters per capita, 1983
ANFAT	Animal fat consumption in calories per capita per day, 1983

For those explanatory variables included in the contemporaneous infant mortality regression, the data are from circa 1990.
SOURCE: OECD (1996) and the authors' calculations.

positively correlated with GDP per capita, especially in the circa 1990 data (table 4–3). Another interesting result is that richer countries have fewer male smokers as a percentage of the male population but more female smokers. (The male and female smoking variables are uncorrelated with a correlation coefficient on the order of −0.01 in both the circa 1983 and the circa 1990 data.) Each of these two correlations is significant. Male life expectancies tend to be positively correlated with income, consumption of animal fat and alcohol (probably again, due to the correlation between alcohol consumption and income) and both pharmaceutical and other health care consumption. Male life expectancies are negatively correlated with

TABLE 4–2

CROSS-CORRELATIONS OF THE VARIABLES INCLUDED IN LIFE EXPECTANCY AND LAGGED INFANT MORTALITY REGRESSIONS

	PHPC	GDPPC	HEPC	MALE SMOKE	FEMALE SMOKE	ALCOHOL	ANFAT
MLE	0.4101	0.6267[a]	0.4952[a]	−0.4097	NA	0.3274	0.5199[b]
MLE40	0.3887	0.5191[b]	0.3460	−0.2277	NA	0.2292	0.2570
MLE60	0.5034[b]	0.4974[b]	0.3135	−0.1540	NA	0.3129	0.1801
FLE	0.5170[b]	0.6296[a]	0.4993[b]	NA	0.0329	0.5142[b]	0.5383[b]
FLE40	0.5989[a]	0.5945[a]	0.4569[b]	NA	−0.0738	0.5065[b]	0.3430
FLE60	0.6122[a]	0.6646[a]	0.5133[b]	NA	0.0113	0.5695[a]	0.4082
INFMORT	−0.4120	−0.6114[a]	−0.4914[b]	NA	−0.1117	−0.4914[b]	−0.6469[a]
PHPC	1.0000	0.3269	0.1887	−0.1124	−0.0876	0.6160[b]	0.2412
GDPPC		1.0000	0.8166[a]	−0.5350[b]	0.4625[b]	0.4055	0.6499[b]
HEPC			1.0000	−0.6320[a]	0.3146	0.1994	0.6226[b]
MALESMOKE				1.0000	NA	−0.1768	−0.4785[b]
FEMALESMOKE					1.0000	−0.0354	0.4280
ALCOHOL						1.0000	0.3926

NOTE: See note to table 4–1.
a. Correlation coefficient significantly different from zero at the 0.01 level.
b. Correlation coefficient significantly different from zero at the 0.05 level.
NA = Not applicable.
SOURCE: OECD (1996) and the authors' calculations.

TABLE 4–3
Cross-Correlations of the Variables Included in the Contemporaneous Infant Mortality Regressions

	PHPC	GDPPC	HEPC	FEMALE SMOKE	ALCOHOL	ANFAT
INFMORT	− 0.3404	− 0.6437[a]	− 0.5078[b]	− 0.0752	− 0.5727[a]	− 0.6130[a]
PHPC	1.0000	0.3076	0.3064	− 0.5348[b]	0.5711[a]	0.2563
GDPPC		1.0000	0.9187[a]	0.2016	0.5527[a]	0.7118[a]
HEPC			1.0000	0.0494	0.5007[b]	0.6410[a]
FEMALESMOKE				1.0000	− 0.2066	0.1653
ALCOHOL					1.0000	0.6339[a]

NOTE: See note to table 4–1.
a. Correlation coefficient significantly different from zero at the 0.01 level.
b. Correlation coefficient significantly different from zero at the 0.05 level.
SOURCE: OECD (1996) and the authors' calculations.

smoking. Female life expectancies follow basically the same pattern except that smoking apparently has no effect on female life expectancies; this outcome most likely occurs because more women smoke in richer countries.

Infant mortality is found to be negatively correlated with GDP per capita, health expenditures per capita, alcohol consumption (again likely due to the positive correlation between alcohol consumption and GDP per capita), and animal fat consumption. This is true whether the explanatory variables are lagged or contemporaneous. Interestingly, infant mortality is not significantly correlated with female smoking rates. This circumstance may indicate that women stop smoking during pregnancy or that smoking causes birth defects but not necessarily an increased chance of infant death. Neither of these possibilities seems particularly likely; the result is most likely caused by correlations with other explanatory variables.

Empirical Results for Life Expectancy

Table 4–4 reports the key empirical results for life expectancy. In these regressions, we analyze life expectancies at birth, at forty years of age, and at sixty years of age for our full sample of twenty-one OECD countries.

Originally, we ran regressions for each sex at each age separately, and the results indicated that observations could be pooled across sexes. To test for this, we pooled observations for each age-specific life expectancy across sexes and included a dummy variable for female life expectancy to allow the intercept to differ by sex. As part of the test, we included interaction terms to allow the slope coefficients to vary by sex. They were not statistically significant as a bloc. The only interaction term that was significant individually in any pooled regression was the interaction of the female dummy and alcohol consumption. We therefore decided to pool across sexes including this interaction. The ln(SMOKE) variable is equal to ln(FEMSMOKE) for those observations on female life ex-

TABLE 4–4
CONSTANT-ELASTICITY REGRESSION RESULTS OF LIFE
EXPECTANCY FOR FULL SAMPLE
(t-statistics in parentheses)

Regressor	At Birth	At Age 40	At Age 60
CONSTANT	− 0.5344[a]	− 0.0256	− 0.8954
	(− 1.7130)	(− 0.0370)	(− 0.8130)
FEMALE	0.0392[b]	0.0996[b]	0.1369[b]
	(4.2480)	(5.4290)	(5.1200)
ln(PHPC)	0.0050	0.0172[a]	0.0401[b]
	(1.0860)	(1.7400)	(2.6950)
ln(GDPPC)	0.0121	0.0572[b]	0.0876[b]
	(0.8310)	(2.1470)	(2.3190)
ln(HEPC)	0.0052	− 0.0111	− 0.0145
	(0.7820)	(− 0.8270)	(− 0.7290)
ln(SMOKE)	− 0.0071	− 0.0102	0.0020
	(− 1.1120)	(− 0.7460)	(0.1020)
ln(ALCOHOL)	− 0.0093[b]	− 0.0143	− 0.0188
	(− 2.3890)	(− 1.6230)	(− 1.3410)
ln(ALCOHOL) X FEMALE	0.0167[b]	0.0150[b]	0.0312[b]
	(4.8500)	(2.1060)	(2.9850)
ln(ANFAT)	1.4040[b]	0.9548[b]	0.9096[b]
	(13.7640)	(4.1660)	(2.5180)
ln(ANFAT)-squared	− 0.1045[b]	− 0.0728[b]	− 0.0706[b]
	(− 13.3550)	(− 4.1710)	(− 2.5690)
R-squared	0.9621	0.9308	0.9290
Adjusted R-squared	0.9515	0.9113	0.9090
Shapiro-Wilkes p-value	0.7068	0.5968	0.5310
Sample size	42	42	42

NOTE: See note to table 4–1.
a. Significant at the 0.10 level based on a two-tailed test.
b. Significant at the 0.05 level based on a two-tailed test.
SOURCE: Authors' model.

pectancy and equal to ln(MALESMOKE) for those observations on male life expectancy.

The Effect of Lifestyle. First, and surprisingly, the lifestyle variable with the greatest apparent effect on life expectancy at all ages is the consumption of animal fat. The results indicate that consumption of animal fat has a strong and large positive effect on all three life expectancy measures at low levels of consumption and this effect is estimated quite precisely. The negative coefficient on the second-order term indicates that this effect falls in magnitude as consumption of animal fat increases and even becomes negative at a high enough level of animal fat intake. This is further evidence of the epidemiological transition; see Gage and O'Connor (1994). At low levels of fat consumption, enriching a diet is beneficial to health, but, at some point, further consumption of fat decreases life expectancy. Excessive fat intake has been linked to degenerative diseases such as heart disease and cancer.

How much animal fat is too much? The results indicate that the effect of animal fat consumption becomes negative for life expectancies at birth, age forty, and age sixty beyond daily consumption levels of 827 calories, 705 calories, and 628 calories, respectively. The caloric consumption measures translate to 92 grams, 78 grams, and 70 grams, respectively. These results are interesting for two reasons. First, given the epidemiological transition, one would expect animal fat to be more helpful at birth than at advanced ages since a rich diet would decrease mortality early in life, when infectious disease is a major killer, but be less effective and more likely to increase mortality at more advanced ages, when degenerative disease becomes important. The detrimental effects of too rich a diet at advanced ages are offset by the positive effects of a rich diet in the early years of life, when we consider life expectancy at birth. When we consider the life expectancies at ages forty and sixty, this positive effect is not as important; we find negative returns to fat consumption at lower levels. The numbers are close to the U.S. Food and Drug Administration's dietary guidelines, which call for fat consumption to be no higher than 80 grams in a 2,500-calorie diet.

The point estimates also indicate that smoking has a small negative effect on life expectancy at birth and at age forty and no effect on life expectancy at age sixty. This, however, is not precisely estimated. The 95 percent confidence interval for the effect of smoking on life expectancy at age sixty includes an elasticity of plus or minus 4 percent.

Alcohol consumption has negative and significant effects on male life expectancy at birth and at age forty, but the slight magnitudes of the effects indicate that doubling alcohol consumption will lower life expectancy only by at most 1.5 percent. This is somewhat surprising, given the epidemiological research showing that moderate drinking (up to three drinks a day) substantially reduces the risk of heart disease (Gaziano et al. 1993). The interactions between alcohol consumption and the female dummy indicate that alcohol consumption has roughly no effect on female life expectancies. This most likely reflects the difference in alcohol consumption between women and men. If men drink most alcohol in all countries, variation in aggregate alcohol consumption will largely be a variation in male alcohol consumption and have a bigger effect on male life expectancy than on female life expectancy. These results are quite different from those found in some previous studies, especially Cochrane, St. Leger, and Moore (1978), which found that cigarette smoking and alcohol consumption are important determinants of mortality.

The Effect of Wealth. Wealth, as measured by lagged gross domestic product per capita, has a positive effect on life expectancy although the effect is significant only for life expectancies at 40 and 60. The results indicate that doubling gross domestic product will increase life expectancy at 40 by roughly 6 percent and life expectancy at 60 by roughly 9 percent. In terms of remaining years of life, a 60-year-old man living in a country with the average life expectancy at 60 could expect to see his remaining life expectancy increase from roughly 18.5 years to roughly 20 years. A 60-year-old female living in such a country could expect to see her remaining life expectancy increase from 22.5 years to roughly 24.5 years.

These are large increases and not terribly surprising since economic growth has been associated with rising life expectancies over the past two centuries. These results are consistent with most previous studies, the most notable exceptions being Auster, Leveson, and Sarachek (1969) and Zweifel and Ferrari (1992).[3] In each of these two studies, increased per capita wealth was associated with higher mortality rates and lower life expectancies, respectively.

The Effect of Nonpharmaceutical Health Care Consumption. The most surprising results relate pharmaceutical consumption and other health care consumption to life expectancy. First, our measure of health care consumption has virtually no effect on life expectancy at birth and is negatively related to life expectancy at the ages of forty and sixty, although the relationship is not statistically significant in any analysis. Further, the negative relationship is weak in terms of magnitudes. The elasticity is never greater in absolute magnitude than -0.0145. Our data reject any large effect of either sign. As pointed out in the literature review, this is not the first study to find a weak negative relationship between life expectancy and health care consumption, especially among developed countries. Cochrane, St. Leger, and Moore (1978), for instance, found a negative relationship, albeit a weak one, between many medical inputs and life expectancy. The result, however, does conflict with Zweifel and Ferrari (1992). Developed countries could be on the flat of the curve for nonpharmaceutical health care consumption, or this result could simply reflect a bias due to the endogeneity of health care consumption and a nation's health.

The Effect of Pharmaceutical Consumption. Pharmaceutical consumption appears surprisingly productive. It has positive and statistically significant relationships with the life expectancies at the ages of 40 and 60. Doubling pharmaceutical expenditures would increase life expectancy at 40 by roughly 2 percent and life expectancy at 60 by about 4 percent. A typical 60-year-old male living in a country with the average life expectancy at age 60, for example, could expect to see his remaining life expectancy rise from 18.5 years to 19.2 years. A typical 60-year-old female living in a country with average life expectancy at age 60 could expect to see her life expectancy rise from 22.5 years to 23.5 years. These results differ sharply from those found in the flawed study by Babazono and Hillman (1994), where pharmaceutical consumption had no significant effect on life expectancy in OECD countries. At the same time, the findings are consistent with the results of Lichtenberg (1996) and others who have found, in microstudies and in studies of restricted formularies, that pharmaceutical consumption is associated with lower mortality rates and better health outcomes.

Table 4–5 presents the marginal effects of drug consumption on the male and female life expectancies at birth, at age forty, and at age sixty. The marginal effects are measured in additional days of life expected per additional 1990 U.S. dollar spent on pharmaceuticals in 1985. The most interesting result is that countries such as France, Italy, Germany, and Belgium—the biggest consumers of drugs—stand to gain the least by marginally increasing their drug consumption. Conversely, the beneficial effect of increased drug consumption is much higher in low—drug-consumption countries such as Ireland, where the effect is roughly five times greater than in France. The results indicate that a country such as Turkey—where drug consumption is extremely low by OECD standards—could dramatically improve life expectancy by increasing pharmaceutical consumption.

The fact that those countries spending the most on pharmaceuticals show the smallest marginal gains in life expectancies is determined by the functional form used in our analysis. The double-log model forces the marginal effect to decrease as pharmaceutical expenditure levels increase. The log-log functional form implies that doubling drug consumption would cut the marginal effect in half. Attempts to test the extent of the flattening of the curve empirically by adding a second-order term for drug use were, as discussed, unsuccessful. The diminishing productivity of drugs (and other inputs) at high use levels makes excellent sense theoretically and fits the data well. We can be less certain of how rapidly diminishing returns set in. Clearly, big spenders on pharmaceuticals such as France, Germany, Italy, and Belgium could cut back on pharmaceutical consumption with less effect on life expectancy than the low spenders such as Turkey, Ireland, and the Netherlands.

Table 4–5 also illustrates that the effect of pharmaceutical consumption on life expectancy, as measured in additional days per dollar spent in 1985, increases with age. The results indicate, for instance, that, in the United States, a dollar spent on pharmaceuticals for a newborn male would increase life expectancy by 0.8 days, a dollar spent on pharmaceuticals for a forty-year-old male would increase life expectancy by 1.4 days, and that same dollar spent on pharmaceuticals for a sixty-year-old male would increase life expectancy by 1.8 days. The same pattern follows in all countries and for both males and females.

The pattern of elasticities does not make this point. The elasticity of remaining life expectancy with respect to pharmaceutical expenditures would be larger for sixty-year-olds than for forty-year-olds simply because remaining life expectancies are shorter at sixty than at forty. To see this consider the formula for the elasticity. It is

TABLE 4–5

MARGINAL EFFECTS OF PHARMACEUTICAL CONSUMPTION ON LIFE EXPECTANCIES AT VARIOUS AGES
(in additional days of life expected)

Country	Females			Males		
	Birth	40	60	Birth	40	60
United States of America	0.784	1.390	1.820	0.719	1.212	1.501
Australia	0.734	1.403	1.841	0.727	1.234	1.515
Austria	0.930	1.644	2.123	0.855	1.423	1.719
Belgium	0.501	0.890	1.159	0.459	0.763	0.912
Canada	0.946	1.704	2.272	0.873	1.488	1.832
Denmark	0.958	1.657	2.119	0.893	1.470	1.743
Finland	0.850	1.563	1.992	0.807	1.320	1.579
France	0.303	0.549	0.734	0.273	0.461	0.579
Germany	0.460	0.810	1.042	0.428	0.697	0.838
Greece	0.682	1.212	1.546	0.639	1.095	1.348

Ireland	1.595	2.743	3.451	1.482	2.427	2.796
Italy	0.447	0.799	1.038	0.412	0.692	0.843
Netherlands	1.131	1.979	2.551	1.046	1.712	2.007
New Zealand	0.575	1.016	1.322	0.533	0.901	1.088
Norway	0.792	1.402	1.813	0.732	1.222	1.457
Portugal	0.813	1.428	1.815	0.738	1.230	1.480
Spain	0.704	1.272	1.661	0.638	1.093	1.354
Sweden	0.712	1.270	1.654	0.665	1.124	1.371
Switzerland	0.872	1.576	2.087	0.800	1.370	1.683
Turkey	4.359	7.891	9.403	4.085	6.949	8.177
United Kingdom	0.935	1.634	2.081	0.872	1.443	1.691

SOURCE: Authors' calculations.

$$\eta = \frac{\partial L}{\partial P} \times \frac{P}{L} \qquad (4\text{--}1)$$

where P is the level of pharmaceutical expenditures and L is the remaining life expectancy. Suppose that the marginal effect on remaining life expectancy of an additional dollar of pharmaceutical spending—the derivative in the formula—were the same both for forty-year-olds and for sixty-year-olds but that the average forty-year-old could expect to live an additional forty years and the average sixty-year-old could expect only to live an additional twenty years. Then the elasticity would be greater for sixty-year-olds simply because L is smaller. By solving for the marginal effect, we find that this is not the only reason why the elasticity is greater for sixty-year-olds but that the marginal effect itself was bigger.

In table 4–6 we present estimates of the lifetime per capita pharmaceutical expenditures made on behalf of forty- and sixty-year-old males and females necessary to extend their lives by one year. The estimates are fairly conservative because they are based on the assumption that pharmaceutical expenditures are constant at 1985 levels over the entire lifetimes of the individuals. These results are highly sensitive to assumptions made about the histories of pharmaceutical consumption in each country.

Expressed in dollars per life year, table 4–6 is commensurate with analyses for new drugs or technologies. The results here tell the same story as in table 4–5. Again, the highest expenditures are necessary in France, Germany, Italy, and Belgium, and the lowest are necessary in Ireland, the Netherlands, and Turkey. The costs are also higher for forty-year-olds than for sixty-year-olds. The magnitudes reflect our conservative assumptions. More realistic assumptions about actual lifetime drug use will lead to lower estimates of cost per life year.

Sensitivity of the Results. To check for the sensitivity of our results to small changes in our model, we tried several

TABLE 4–6
LIFETIME COST OF EXTENDING LIFE BY
ONE YEAR AT AGES FORTY AND SIXTY
(in 1990 U.S. $)

Country	Females		Males	
	Forty	Sixty	Forty	Sixty
United States	21,165	16,607	22,707	19,167
Australia	21,358	16,591	22,729	19,152
Austria	17,936	14,198	19,320	16,621
Belgium	33,293	26,147	36,034	31,264
Canada	17,670	13,545	18,917	15,857
Denmark	17,406	14,020	18,527	16,251
Finland	18,826	15,061	20,542	17,934
France	55,127	42,081	60,226	50,081
Germany	36,303	28,853	39,246	33,989
Greece	24,486	19,500	25,778	21,585
Ireland	10,527	8,578	11,219	10,063
Italy	37,462	29,333	40,273	34,220
Netherlands	14,884	11,806	16,036	14,134
New Zealand	28,917	22,807	30,758	26,370
Norway	21,160	16,691	22,693	19,646
Portugal	20,400	16,431	22,040	19,158
Spain	23,662	18,409	25,547	21,399
Sweden	23,539	18,410	25,026	21,141
Switzerland	19,171	14,746	20,566	17,263
Turkey	3,515	3,043	3,766	3,393
United Kingdom	17,890	14,367	19,077	16,791

SOURCE: Authors' calculations.

variants. We reestimated the models and excluded Turkey because Turkey is quite different from the rest of the countries in our sample in such key measures as wealth, pharmaceutical consumption, and life expectancy. Male life expectancy at birth in Turkey, for instance, was 65.4 years in 1993, whereas the next lowest life expectancy was Portugal's, at 70.8 years. Since ordinary least squares estimators can be sensitive to such outliers, one might fear that the observations for Turkey were driving the results.

The exclusion of Turkey from the analysis did not significantly change the results. The elasticity of pharmaceutical consumption, for instance, was 0.016 (instead of 0.017) for life expectancy at age 40 and equal to 0.039 (instead of 0.040) for life expectancy at age 60. These estimates were significant at the same levels as in the inclusive regressions reported in table 4–4. Therefore, including Turkey does not drive the results.

We also ran regressions after restricting the sample to the European countries. Table 4–7 reports the results. They are similar to those from our original inclusive regressions, although some differences emerge. First, pharmaceutical consumption has a larger and more statistically significant positive effect for Europe than in our original sample, which also included Turkey, North America, and Oceania. Second, the effect of wealth is smaller and insignificant. If anything, pharmaceutical consumption is even more productive in producing health in Europe than it is elsewhere.

As an additional test for sensitivity, the lifestyle variables were dropped from the models. Excluding the lifestyle variables, the positive effect of pharmaceutical consumption is much greater for all three life expectancies, especially at the younger ages. The effect of wealth is greatly increased in the regression for life expectancy at birth but not at later ages. Finally, the effect of other health care consumption does not change in any appreciable way. Apparently, controlling for lifestyle factors is important to avoid overstating the beneficial effect of pharmaceutical consumption on health.

We included other factors that may help determine life expectancy. None appears satisfactory. A variable equal to the natural log of the percentage of the population aged sixty-five and older, for instance, was included to investigate the endogeneity of spending argument: since the elderly tend to use more drugs and, at the same time, their presence also drives up life expectancy measures, the positive effect of pharmaceutical consumption

TABLE 4–7

CONSTANT-ELASTICITY REGRESSION RESULTS
OF LIFE EXPECTANCY FOR EUROPEAN COUNTRIES

(*t*-statistics in parentheses)

Regressor	At Birth	At Age 40	At Age 60
CONSTANT	−0.8722	−4.2760[a]	−5.9190
	(−0.9360)	(−1.9060)	(−1.5420)
FEMALE	0.0460[b]	0.0808[b]	0.1393[b]
	(3.9620)	(3.4870)	(3.7130)
ln(PHPC)	0.0090[a]	0.0230[b]	0.0501[b]
	(1.9110)	(2.3370)	(3.2100)
ln(GDPPC)	0.0094	0.0228	0.0353[b]
	(0.4920)	(0.5080)	(0.5160)
ln(HEPC)	0.0020	−0.0059	−0.0083
	(0.2600)	(−0.3360)	(−0.3070)
ln(SMOKE)	−0.0104	−0.0096	0.0055
	(−1.4910)	(−0.6950)	(0.2840)
ln(ALCOHOL)	−0.0090[b]	−0.0118	−0.0108
	(−2.2710)	(−1.3220)	(−0.6410)
ln(ALCOHOL)	0.0132[b]	0.0238[b]	0.0324[a]
X FEMALE	(2.7100)	(2.3160)	(1.9120)
ln(ANFAT)	1.5010[b]	2.2700[b]	2.4860[a]
	(4.9460)	(3.1270)	(2.0250)
ln(ANFAT)-	−0.1107[b]	−0.1687[b]	−0.1858[a]
squared	(−4.9520)	(−3.1480)	(−2.0440)
R-squared	0.9574	0.9386	0.9350
Adjusted *R*-squared	0.9400	0.9135	0.9084
Shapiro-Wilkes			
p-value	0.6668	0.8728	0.3420
Sample size	32	32	32

a. Significant at the 0.10 level based on a two-tailed test.
b. Significant at the 0.05 level based on a two-tailed test.
SOURCE: Authors' model.

in our regressions may be due to an omitted variable bias. The effect of the variable that we included was insignificant and tended to dampen the GDP effect and strengthen the drug consumption effect in every regression. The coefficient on this variable was also negative. These results contradict the endogeneity of spending argument and indicate that pharmaceutical consumption drives up life expectancies even when controlling for the aged population.

We also included variables for mean years of education and unemployment. Neither of these variables was significant in any of the regressions, and the effects of the other variables remained the same. For education, this could be due to the fact that twelve years of education, for example, likely means different things in the different countries considered here.

We also replaced our smoking variables with an alternative measure: the natural log of the daily consumption of tobacco in grams per capita. The results were curious, as this version of the smoking variable had a slight positive effect on life expectancy. This was even further from our expectations. Also, the effect of drug consumption increased slightly. We prefer measuring smoking as the percentage of the adult population who smoke: most health researchers believe that the adverse effects of smoking begin at low levels of consumption. The effect of switching from ten cigarettes a day to two packs a day is small, but the effect of switching from being a nonsmoker to smoking ten cigarettes a day is huge. The percentage of the population who smoke captures this inherent nonlinearity better than the consumption of tobacco, averaged across the entire population.

Finally, we replaced our measure of pharmaceutical consumption with one constructed by converting expenditures to U.S. dollars with the GDP purchasing power parity exchange rates. In each model, the elasticity for pharmaceutical consumption fell substantially and was never significant. For the reasons stated, this measure of pharmaceutical consumption is inferior to the one used in this study.

Empirical Results for Infant Mortality

Table 4–8 presents results from the analysis of infant mortality based on two constant-elasticity regressions. In the first one, contemporaneous levels of the regressors explain infant mortality in 1990. The second regression explains infant mortality by values of the regressors that have been lagged by five to seven years (as in the life expectancy regressions). We do this for two reasons. First, the a priori case for lagged regressors in explaining infant mortality is not as strong as for life expectancy. Second, unlike life expectancy, the choice of contemporaneous or lagged regressors makes a major difference in the results.

The Effect of Lifestyle. Lifestyle factors make a big difference for infant mortality. In both regressions reported in table 4–8, one can reject the hypothesis that all four lifestyle coefficients are zero. The nutrition variable—the amount of animal fat calories consumed per capita per day—is significantly negatively related to infant mortality in both regressions, although the positive coefficient on the second-order term indicates that the beneficial effects of increased animal fat consumption diminish as more and more is consumed. Animal fat consumption actually becomes harmful at consumption levels above 1,053 calories in the contemporaneous regression and above 965 calories in the lagged regression. The beneficial effect of animal fat consumption, at least at levels below 1,000 calories per day, is again consistent with the idea of the epidemiological transition. Those diseases most likely to kill infants are those for which a rich diet is most helpful. The bad effects of a diet that is too rich would most likely be due to issues pertaining to maternal behavior at the prenatal stage. Extremely rich diets are probably correlated

TABLE 4–8
CONSTANT-ELASTICITY REGRESSION RESULTS FOR
INFANT MORTALITY IN 1990
(*t*-statistics in parentheses)

Regressor	Contemporaneous	Lagged Five Years
CONSTANT	53.7210[a]	51.3900[a]
	(11.4630)	(17.2250)
ln(PHPC)	0.0026	0.0753
	(0.0300)	(1.5610)
ln(GDPPC)	− 0.4943	0.0307
	(− 1.7900)	(0.1880)
ln(HEPC)	0.1642	− 0.1899[a]
	(0.9770)	(− 3.2360)
ln(FEMSMOKE)	− 0.0294	0.1654
	(− 0.1460)	(1.6690)
ln(ALCOHOL)	− 0.0233	− 0.0246
	(− 0.2670)	(− 0.6970)
ln(ANFAT)	− 13.8000[a]	− 14.3500[a]
	(− 9.5890)	(− 13.7700)
ln(ANFAT)-squared	0.9915[a]	1.0440[a]
	(9.4370)	(12.9110)
R-squared	0.9436	0.9659
Adjusted *R*-squared	0.9132	0.9475
Shapiro-Wilkes *p*-value	0.3814	0.1493
Sample size	21	21

a. Significant at the 0.05 level based on a two-tailed test.
SOURCE: Authors' model.

with other behavioral characteristics that we have not directly controlled for, such as maternal obesity or diabetes.

The results for smoking are more problematic. In the contemporaneous regression, female smoking appears to have a small negative and statistically insignificant effect on infant mortality. The result is imprecise. At the 95 percent level, for instance, we could not reject a positive effect of nearly 0.20. Though imprecise, this result differs from most previous studies, including the one by Cochrane, St. Leger, and Moore (1978). In the lagged regression, female smoking has a strong, marginally statistically significant positive effect on infant mortality, a result consistent with previous studies. While the more reasonable result from the better-fitting lagged regression is comforting, the result from the contemporaneous regression is troubling because of the general belief that smoking during pregnancy leads to birth defects and low birth weight. Perhaps there is a subtle selection problem here. Smoking during pregnancy may lead to poorer fetal health and thus more miscarriages and stillbirths. But perhaps there is not much effect on infant mortality for those fetuses that survive to a live birth. The results on alcohol consumption are not mixed. In both regressions, alcohol consumption has a slight negative, although statistically insignificant, association with infant mortality.

The Effect of Wealth. The results on the effects of wealth on infant mortality are mixed. Gross domestic product per capita has the expected negative effect on infant mortality in the contemporaneous regression. In the lagged regression, however, it has a small, insignificant positive effect on infant mortality. The results in the contemporaneous model indicate that a doubling of gross domestic product per capita would cut infant mortality by nearly 50 percent. The average country would see a fall in infant mortality from roughly ten infant deaths to only five infant deaths per 1,000 live births. The results in the lagged regression indicate that, for the average country, a doubling of the gross domestic product would slightly increase infant mortality, by roughly 3 percent. Again, this effect is imprecisely measured. Our data cannot reject a negative effect as large as -0.16 at the 95 percent level.

The Effect of Nonpharmaceutical Health Care Consumption. Again, the results on the effect of nonpharmaceutical health care are mixed. In the contemporaneous regression, the effect is positive and insignificant, whereas the effect is negative and significant in the lagged regression. The result from the contemporaneous regression is much like the one found by Cochrane, St. Leger, and Moore (1978), who found that the number of doctors per capita in general, and of pediatricians per capita in particular, has a positive (harmful) effect on infant mortality. The result from the lagged regression is similar to the one found by some others, particularly Hadley (1982). The result from the lagged regression indicates that doubling health care consumption would lower infant mortality in the average country from roughly ten deaths per 1,000 live births to roughly eight deaths per 1,000 live births.

The Effect of Pharmaceutical Consumption. In each regression, pharmaceutical consumption per capita has a small positive effect on infant mortality. The effect is slight and not significant in the contemporaneous regression, while it is larger and marginally significant in the lagged regression, where the t-statistic is 1.56. The point estimate would seem to indicate that after controlling for wealth, other health care consumption, and lifestyle factors, increased pharmaceutical consumption may actually increase infant mortality, although the contemporaneous regression results indicate that pharmaceutical consumption has no effect on infant mortality. The result is not precise. Given the usual standard for statistical inference, we cannot rule out the possibility that there is as much as a 2 percent negative effect of pharmaceutical consumption on infant mortality.

A small effect of pharmaceutical consumption on infant mortality makes sense in light of the results from the regressions for life expectancy. Pharmaceutical consumption apparently has great potential for extending life in one's later years, but it can do little to improve the likelihood of survival for the young. For the young, nutrition plays a much larger role. Also, the pharmaceutical consumption variable is the average pharmaceutical expenditures for the entire population. Data on the pharmaceutical consumption of infants or women during pregnancy are not available.

Sensitivity of the Results. The sensitivity of our results was checked in the same manner as they were for the life expectancy regression results. Excluding Turkey from the analysis did not change the results in the lagged regression in any appreciable way. In the contemporaneous regression, no individual variables were statistically significant after Turkey was dropped, not even the variables for richness of diet. Further, dropping North America and Oceania and leaving only the sixteen European countries changed the results somewhat in the contemporaneous regression. For one, the effect of smoking became positive and marginally significant (at the 25 percent level). The effect of pharmaceutical consumption became more positive with an elasticity of 0.08 but was estimated imprecisely. The effect of wealth became more negative with an elasticity of -0.8441 but was less precisely measured. In the lagged regression, the effects of wealth and alcohol consumption both went from being positive and insignificant to being negative and insignificant.

We dropped the lifestyle variables from our analysis as an additional test for sensitivity. Here the results on pharmaceutical consumption are quite different. The effect of pharmaceutical consumption is negative in each regression and is significant in the lagged regression, where the elasticity is -0.32. The effect of wealth is large, negative (the elasticity is -1.5), and significant in the contemporaneous regression (no doubt capturing a good deal of the effect of nutrition). It is also negative, though much smaller and insignificant, in the lagged regression. Finally, the effect of health care consumption changes but not in a significant way. It remains positive and insignificant in the contemporaneous regression and negative and significant in the lagged regression.

The infant mortality model was much less successful than the life expectancy models. Most results are sensitive to small, and perfectly defensible, changes to our model. The infant mortality results must be counted as suggestive at best.

5

Conclusion

The purpose of this analysis has been to study the production of health with emphasis on the productivity of pharmaceutical consumption and other health care. Whereas pharmaceutical consumption has been shown to have a positive effect on health in micro-studies and in studies of restricted formularies, such an effect has not previously been found in studies of international aggregate data. But such studies are rare and are usually flawed. Most cross-national work, driven by an obsession with cost-containment, has concentrated on expenditures rather than on health.

Results have been mixed on the effects of wealth and general health expenditures on health outcomes in the few international studies of the production of health. Most such studies have found that lifestyle and environmental factors have a much greater impact than health care, especially in the developing world, but also among developed countries.

Many of these studies, however, have been flawed. Some have used poor measures of health care inputs and have transformed national expenditures to common units by using inappropriate price measures. Others have used measures such as the number of hospital beds or hospital lengths of stay and compared them across countries although such comparisons are most likely inappropriate. Hospitals serve different functions in different countries; comparing hospital statistics across countries is particularly unenlightening. Finally, few studies have taken account of the fact that the production of health exhibits diminishing returns; thus few have used functional forms that allow for such diminishing returns.

In this study, we have estimated a production function for health that is a function of pharmaceutical consumption, other health care consumption, gross domestic product, and three lifestyle measures: alcohol consumption, the percentage of the population who smoke, and the richness of diet. Purchasing power parity exchange rates for pharmaceuticals and health care were used to transform pharmaceutical expenditures and health care expenditures to U.S. dollars. The dependent variables were life expectancies at birth, at age forty, and at age sixty and infant mortality.

In a sample of twenty-one OECD countries, pharmaceutical consumption has a positive and significant (both statistically and economically) effect on remaining life expectancy at age forty and at age sixty. It has a small, positive, and statistically insignificant effect on life expectancy at birth. The elasticities of pharmaceutical consumption on life expectancy are roughly 0.017 at age forty and 0.040 at age sixty. The estimates are not sensitive to small changes in the basic statistical models. In a sample of only the sixteen European countries for which complete data are available, these elasticities are higher (0.023 for age forty and 0.050 for age sixty), and pharmaceutical consumption had a small positive significant effect on life expectancy at birth.

No significant effect of pharmaceutical consumption on infant mortality was found. Taken at face value, one model even suggests that, in controlling for lifestyle factors, increased pharmaceutical consumption may be related to slightly increased infant mortality. Unfortunately, the sensitivity of results of the infant mortality model to small changes does not inspire much confidence in infant mortality as a health output measure, at least not in this data set. This measurement problem also affects life expectancy at birth to some extent.

We found the gross domestic product to have a positive and significant effect on life expectancies at the ages of forty and sixty, although this effect is not present in the European-only sample. The results from the infant mortality regressions are mixed. We found no effect of non-pharmaceutical health care consumption in any of the life expectancy regressions. We did find, however, a negative effect on infant mortality in one specification.

The lifestyle variable with the biggest effect on health is dietary richness, as measured by the consumption of animal fat. Increased richness of diet improves mortality up to a point, but the impact becomes negative as a diet becomes very rich. This result is consistent with the epidemiological transition: the idea that, at low nutritional levels, enriching a diet allows one to better fight off infections but that, at high nutritional levels, enriching a diet leads to a greater incidence of degenerative diseases such as cancer and heart disease. Still, this is a slightly surprising result since most researchers might think that the OECD countries are wealthy enough that nutrition, in this basic sense, should not be an issue.

This study should add to the debate over how OECD governments should allocate scarce medical care resources. It improves on much of the existing literature since it uses better measures of pharmaceutical and other health care consumption and uses a functional form that allows for diminishing returns. The results have been surprising, but they have also been fairly robust. Increased pharmaceutical consumption helps improve mortality outcomes, especially for those at middle age and beyond.

An Attempt at Duplicating Zweifel and Ferrari's (1992) Results

A n attempt was made to duplicate the results of Peter Zweifel and Matteo Ferrari (1992) with the 1996 OECD heath data because the results of our study do not coincide with Zweifel and Ferrari's. Specifically, in lagged regressions similar to ours, Zweifel and Ferrari found that gross domestic product per capita has a negative effect on life expectancies at the ages of forty and sixty-five and that general health expenditures have a significant and positive effect on these life expectancies. We found that per capita gross domestic product has a positive effect on life expectancies at the ages of forty and sixty and that general health expenditures have no measurable effect. But the studies are not identical. Our study, for example, examined data from a different period, the early 1990s, instead of 1980, and it also included countries that were not included in Zweifel and Ferrari's analysis. We used a double-log specification rather than a linear specification and used different conversion factors to convert health expenditures to U.S. dollars.

To learn how our findings differ, we attempted to run the exact same regression that Zweifel and Ferrari report on page 316 of their study, where they regress various life expectancies in 1980 on per capita health expenditures and per capita gross domestic product figures from 1970. The expenditure and gross domestic product figures were converted to U.S. dollars by using gross domestic product purchasing power parity conversions and were left in 1970 dollars. The only difference was our use of life expectancy at age sixty rather than at age sixty-five for the regression since we found availability of data for life expectancy at age sixty-five to be rather spotty (for instance, it is not available for Canada for the years around 1980). The means and extreme values of the variables included in our study and in Zweifel and Ferrari's study are presented in table A–1.

The gross domestic product and health expenditure measures are measured in thousands of U.S. dollars. Since life expectancy at age sixty is used in our analysis, the other variables would not be directly comparable. We do find the extremes for female life expectancy at age sixty to be the same as Zweifel and Ferrari found (Ireland, low; Iceland, high). For males, life expectancy at age sixty was highest in Iceland in our data, whereas it was highest at age sixty-five in Japan in Zweifel and Ferrari's data. Ireland had the lowest male life expectancy at age sixty in our data and also had the lowest life expectancy at age sixty-five in Zweifel and Ferrari's.

Table A–1 also presents the regression results side by side. The results are quite different, although we have attempted to duplicate Zweifel and Ferrari's results exactly here. A conversation with Professor Zweifel led us to believe that, as we had suspected, the difference in the outcomes may result from revisions that the OECD has made to its gross domestic product purchasing power parity exchange rates since 1986. If true, then the results of international studies may be sensitive to revisions made by the OECD and other international data collection organizations.

TABLE A–1
Comparisons with Zweifel and Ferrari

A. Means and Extreme Values

Variable	Our Study			Zweifel and Ferrari		
	Mean	Minimum	Maximum	Mean	Minimum	Maximum
GDP, 1970	3.159	1.782 (Greece)	4.708 (U.S.)	3.512	1.756 (Greece)	4.976 (Sweden)
Health expenditures, 1970	0.175	0.060 (Greece)	0.341 (U.S.)	0.208	0.070 (Greece)	0.366 (U.S.)
Female life expectancy at 40	39.500	36.200 (Ireland)	41.000 (Iceland)	39.500	36.200 (Ireland)	41.600 (Iceland)
Male life expectancy at 40	33.900	31.800 (Finland)	36.400 (Iceland)	33.900	31.800 (Finland)	36.500 (Iceland)

(continued)

67

TABLE A-1 (continued)

B. Regression Results

Variable	Our Study	Zweifel and Ferrari
Intercept	33.40[a]	34.80[a]
Age 65	—.—	−20.70[a]
Age 60	−17.30[a]	—.—
Female	4.90[a]	4.80[a]
GDP, 1970	0.30	−0.88[b]
Health expenditures, 1970	−0.63	12.40[c]
Adjusted R-square	0.98	0.99

a. Significant at the .10 level.
b. Significant at the .01 level.
c. Significant at the .05 level.
SOURCE: Authors' model and Zweifel and Ferrari (1992).

The Data Used in the Analyses in This Study

T he tables in this appendix contain the data set used in the analyses in the main body of the report. Table B–1 presents the dependent variables from the life expectancy regressions. Table B–2 gives the explanatory variables from the life expectancy regressions. These same explanatory variables were used in the lagged infant mortality regression. Table B–3 presents the 1990 infant mortality measures and the explanatory variables from the contemporaneous infant mortality regression. Table B–4 gives cross-correlations among the dependent variables included in the analysis.

The following should be noted about the data used. The life expectancy data in table B–1 are for the year 1993, except for the following cases. For Canada and New Zealand, the data in table B–1 are for the year 1992; for Turkey, the life expectancies are for the year 1990.

In table B–2, the data for pharmaceutical consumption, nonpharmaceutical health care consumption, and gross domestic product are for the year 1985. The other data in table B–2 are for 1983 except for the following cases. For France and for Greece, the smoking data are for the year 1987; for Austria, for the year 1986; and for Germany, for the year 1985. For Ireland, the male smoking data are for 1985 and the female smoking data point is the average of the female smoking variable in 1980 and

TABLE B–1
LIFE EXPECTANCIES FOR SAMPLE COUNTRIES, 1993

Country	MLE	MLE40	MLE60	FLE	FLE40	FLE60
United States	72.2	35.4	18.8	78.8	40.6	22.8
Australia	75.0	37.2	19.5	80.9	42.1	23.7
Austria	73.0	35.3	18.3	79.4	40.8	22.6
Belgium	73.0	35.3	18.1	79.8	41.2	23.0
Canada	74.9	37.1	19.6	81.2	42.5	24.3
Denmark	72.3	34.6	17.6	77.6	39.0	21.4
Finland	72.1	34.3	17.6	79.5	40.6	22.2
France	73.3	36.0	19.4	81.4	42.9	24.6
Germany	73.8	34.9	18.0	79.3	40.6	22.4
Greece	74.9	37.3	19.7	79.9	41.3	22.6

Ireland	72.7	34.6	17.1	78.2	39.1	21.1
Italy	74.5	36.4	19.0	80.9	42.0	23.4
Netherlands	74.0	35.2	17.7	80.0	40.7	22.5
New Zealand	73.1	35.9	18.6	78.9	40.5	22.6
Norway	74.2	36.0	18.4	80.2	41.3	22.9
Portugal	70.8	34.3	17.7	78.0	39.8	21.7
Spain	73.3	36.5	19.4	80.9	42.5	23.8
Sweden	75.5	37.1	19.4	80.8	41.9	23.4
Switzerland	74.7	37.2	19.6	81.4	42.8	24.3
Turkey	64.1	31.7	16.0	68.4	36.0	18.4
United Kingdom	73.6	35.4	17.8	78.9	40.1	21.9

SOURCE: OECD (1996) health data.

TABLE B–2
EXPLANATORY VARIABLES FROM LIFE EXPECTANCY REGRESSIONS

Country	PHPC	GDPPC	HEPC	FEMSMOKE	MALESMOKE	ALCOHOL	ANFAT
United States	183.37	19,876.53	1,935.21	35.1	37.6	10.2	1,192
Australia	188.38	15,683.88	1,131.69	30.9	40.3	12.3	632
Austria	155.78	14,971.05	1,539.26	21.3	40.0	12.6	1,324
Belgium	290.55	14,585.32	1,546.43	27.5	47.0	13.8	1,250
Canada	156.57	17,463.52	1,909.72	28.3	34.0	10.9	1,274
Denmark	147.80	15,895.33	1,075.66	42.5	53.5	12.8	1,245
Finland	163.11	14,283.96	1,471.19	17.0	33.0	7.9	1,170
France	490.68	15,780.17	1,465.85	29.0	43.4	19.1	1,206
Germany	314.53	16,378.13	1,401.59	27.0	41.0	14.3	1,253
Greece	213.95	8,716.64	318.43	25.0	61.0	2.3	817

Ireland	89.50	9,231.58	838.69	30.5	37.0	8.0	1,309
Italy	330.03	14,389.36	890.57	17.7	45.6	12.6	815
Netherlands	129.11	14,474.72	1,659.75	34.0	50.0	10.9	1,168
New Zealand	250.23	13,683.13	873.96	31.2	34.5	10.6	1,156
Norway	184.89	16,995.37	1,716.46	32.0	42.0	4.9	880
Portugal	175.00	7,456.35	547.94	9.0	41.0	13.4	497
Spain	209.66	9,787.78	513.05	20.0	59.0	14.5	825
Sweden	207.13	15,959.31	2,335.83	26.4	31.8	6.1	1,059
Switzerland	170.45	19,667.08	1,374.24	28.0	43.3	13.6	1,192
Turkey	28.64	4,080.08	141.36	24.3	62.8	1.2	252
United Kingdom	154.05	13,983.11	962.12	32.5	37.0	8.7	1,039

Source: OECD (1996) health data.

TABLE B–3
Data Set for Contemporaneous Infant Mortality Regression

Country	INFMORT	PHPC	GDPPC	HEPC	FEMSMOKE	ALCOHOL	ANFAT
United States	9.2	531.00	21,163.00	2,458.00	22.8	9.6	967
Australia	8.2	196.39	15,938.85	1,244.56	27.0	10.3	642
Austria	7.8	191.94	16,599.57	1,638.25	20.3	12.6	1,249
Belgium	8.0	304.47	16,318.33	1,573.48	26.0	12.4	1,148
Canada	6.8	215.65	18,346.15	1,693.91	26.9	9.2	1,188
Denmark	7.5	112.85	16,553.57	1,054.01	40.3	11.6	1,276
Finland	5.6	190.66	16,202.98	1,286.40	21.0	9.5	1,220
France	7.3	560.93	17,357.79	1,704.33	19.2	16.7	1,222
Germany	7.1	374.14	18,351.20	1,369.82	22.2	13.8	1,327
Greece	9.7	216.03	9,132.78	357.19	26.0	2.3	735

Ireland	8.2	120.69	11,239.13	739.31	29.0	9.0	759
Italy	8.2	448.20	16,285.52	1,274.37	17.3	10.9	694
Netherlands	7.1	130.19	15,920.28	1,578.10	31.0	9.9	1,061
New Zealand	8.4	194.83	13,475.78	1,048.58	27.3	10.1	1,034
Norway	7.0	216.34	17,498.46	1,333.46	34.0	5.0	830
Portugal	11.0	247.09	9,375.29	529.35	12.0	9.8	662
Spain	7.6	286.62	11,754.58	806.90	21.4	13.6	792
Sweden	6.0	225.86	17,011.03	1,593.58	25.9	6.4	1,052
Switzerland	6.8	190.48	21,263.64	1,685.12	29.0	12.9	1,162
Turkey	59.3	62.11	4,690.53	163.10	24.3	0.5	276
United Kingdom	7.9	183.72	15,935.00	1,182.95	29.0	8.9	750

SOURCE: OECD (1996) health data.

TABLE B–4
CROSS-CORRELATIONS AMONG DEPENDENT VARIABLES

	INFMORT	MLE	MLE40	MLE60	FLE	FLE40	FLE60
INFMORT	1.0000	−0.3864	−0.6742	−0.5666	−0.9243	−0.7259	−0.7368
MLE		1.0000	0.8934	0.7629	0.9422	0.8370	0.8238
MLE40			1.0000	0.9480	0.8510	0.8925	0.8752
MLE60				1.0000	0.7855	0.9073	0.9004
FLE					1.0000	0.9277	0.9217
FLE40						1.0000	0.9887

NOTE: All correlation coefficients are significantly different from zero at the 0.01 level.
SOURCE: OECD (1996) and authors' calculations.

1986. For Spain, the smoking data are for the year 1982. For Switzerland, the smoking data are weighted averages of the data for the years 1981 and 1987. For Turkey, the smoking data are for the year 1989. For the United Kingdom, the smoking data are the averages of the data for the years 1982 and 1984.

In table B–3, the data are all for the year 1990, with the following exceptions. First, the animal fat data are almost all for the year 1988. The only animal fat data for the year 1990 are the data points for Australia, New Zealand, and Portugal. For Australia, Germany, Spain, and Turkey, the smoking data are for the year 1989; for Austria, for 1991; for Italy, for 1986; and for Portugal, for 1988. Finally, for Greece and for Turkey, the alcohol consumption data reflect consumption in 1989; for the United States, for 1987; and for the United Kingdom, for 1991.

Notes

Chapter 1: Introduction

1. We do not provide a detailed review of this literature since it is not the focus of our research. We do direct interested readers to papers by Joseph Newhouse (1977); David Parkin, Alistair McGuire, and Brian Yule (1987); and Ulf-G Gerdtham and B. Jonsson (1991, 1992).

Chapter 2: A Review of the Literature

1. The sample was limited to whites, mostly because of the sample size.

2. County groups are defined by the Census Bureau and, in 1970, consisted of one or more whole counties with a minimum population of 250,000 people. The county groups are built to conform to local economic and market patterns. An individual county group can encompass counties in more than one state. As of 1970 more than 400 county groups were defined by the Census Bureau.

3. For 1980, county groups were much larger, consisting of one or more whole counties with a minimum population of 1 million.

4. This approach follows Rodgers (1979) and flows from the general idea of diminishing returns to income in the production of health.

5. Also, as we find in sensitivity testing, using the GDP prices (which amounts to ignoring the differences in drug prices relative to other goods across countries) leads to inferior results.

Chapter 3: Data and Methodological Issues

1. See Garattini and colleagues (1994) for an excellent comparison of the pharmaceutical markets and price regulation in Italy, France, Germany, and the United Kingdom.

2. The Fisher price index is the geometric mean of the Laspeyres and Paasche price indexes. Like both the Laspeyres and Paasche indexes, it is intransitive. The product of the indexes, for example, between the United States and Canada and between Canada and Denmark is not equal to the index between the United States and Denmark. Unlike the other two indexes, the Fisher price index yields results that are invariant to which country is used as a base.

3. Other dimensions of health are nearly impossible to measure objectively. These include the level of comfort and the general issue of the quality, as well as length, of life. The availability of these measures tends to be rather spotty even for the OECD countries, and the quality of these measures is yet to be determined. Thus, we focus on life expectancy.

Chapter 4: The Analysis

1. Michael Grossman (1972a, b) did the seminal work on the household production of health.

2. Other specifications were considered. A linear specification was rejected since it would not allow for diminishing returns. Second-order linear specifications were estimated, and the results confirmed the importance of diminishing returns. The estimated residuals from the regressions were highly skewed, and, by using a Shapiro-Wilk test (1965), we could reject the hypothesis that they were normally distributed. Also, multicollinearity was a major problem.

Second-order double logarithmic specifications were also tried, and they were preferable according to Hausman specification tests, but so much multicollinearity was introduced that the results were uninterpretable. Condition indexes from these regressions were in the range of 15,000, which indicated severe multicollinearity. Conventionally, an index of 45 indicates a serious problem; see Greene (1993). Ultimately, a second-order logarithmic term for animal fat calories was included because we did not want to constrain the effect to be monotonic. This also introduced a fair amount of collinearity but improved general model performance.

Adding additional second-order terms did not improve the model's performance. Most important, when we included a squared term for the natural log of pharmaceutical consumption, the collinearity was so extreme that the model was uninterpretable. While diminishing returns to pharmaceutical use (as well as other variables) make theoretical sense and improve model performance significantly, we are not able to use a flexible form to determine the precise shape of the curve depicting diminishing returns; rather, it is determined by the log-log functional form.

3. We also attempted to replicate Zweifel and Ferrari (1992) in detail. See the appendix.

References

Anand, Sudhir, and Martin Ravallion. 1993. "Human Development in Poor Countries: On the Role of Private Incomes and Public Services." *Journal of Economic Perspectives* 7 (1) (winter): 133–50.

———. 1996. "Human Development and Income Growth in Developing Countries: Reply." *Journal of Economic Perspectives* 10 (2) (spring): 210–12.

Auster, Richard, Irving Leveson, and Deborah Sarachek. 1969. "The Production of Health, an Exploratory Study." *Journal of Human Resources* 4 (4) (fall): 411–36.

Babazono, Akira, and Alan L. Hillman. 1994. "A Comparison of International Health Outcomes and Health Care Spending." *International Journal of Technology Assessment in Health Care* 10 (3) (summer): 81.

Baily, Martin Neil, and Alan M. Garber. 1998. "Health Care Productivity." Brookings Papers on Economic Activity: Microeconomics, 1997. Washington, D.C.: Brookings Institution, pp. 143–215.

Cochrane, A. L., A. S. St. Leger, and F. Moore. 1978. "Health Service 'Input' and Mortality 'Output' in Developed Countries." *Journal of Epidemiology and Community Health* 32 (3) (September): 200–205.

Cutler, David, Mark McClellan, and Joseph Newhouse. 1997. "The Costs and Benefits of Intensive Treatment for Cardiovascular Disease." Paper presented at AEI-Brookings Conference on Measuring the Prices of Medical Treatments, December 12.

Danzon, Patricia M., and Allison Percy. 1995. "The Effects of Price Regulation on Productivity in Pharmaceuticals." Unpublished paper, Wharton School, University of Pennsylvania.

Economist. 1996. "The Overprescription Machine." October 19, p. 66.

Fuchs, Victor R. 1974. *Who Shall Live?* New York: Basic Books.

Gage, Timothy B., and Kathleen O'Connor. 1994. "Nutrition and the Variation in Level and Age Patterns of Mortality." *Human Biology* 66 (1) (February): 77–103.

Garattini, Livio, Franco Salvioni, Diego Scopelliti, and Silvio Garattini. 1994. "A Comparative Analysis of the Pharmaceutical Market in Four European Countries." *PharmacoEconomics* 6 (5): 417–23.

Gaziano, J. Michael, Julie E. Buring, Jan L. Breslow, Samuel Z. Goldhaber, Bernard Rosner, Martin VanDenburgh, Walter Willett, and Charles Hennekens. 1993. "Moderate Alcohol Intake, Increased Levels of High-Density Lipoprotein and Its Subfractions, and Decreased Risk of Myocardial Infarction." *New England Journal of Medicine* 329(25) (December 16): 1829–34.

Gerdtham, Ulf-G, and B. Jonsson. 1991. "Price and Quantity in International Comparisons of Health Expenditures." *Applied Economics* 23: 1519–28.

―――. 1992. "An Econometric Analysis of Health Care Expenditure: A Cross-Section Study of the OECD Countries." *Journal of Health Economics* 11: 63–84.

Grabowski, Henry. 1988. "Medicaid Patients' Access to New Drugs." *Health Affairs* 7 (5) (winter): 102–14.

Greene, William H. 1993. *Econometric Analysis.* 2d ed. New York: Macmillan.

Grossman, Michael. 1972a. *The Demand for Health: A Theoretical and Empirical Investigation.* New York: Columbia University Press.

―――. 1972b. "On the Concept of Health Capital and the Demand for Health." *Journal of Political Economy* 80 (2) (April): 223–55.

Hadley, Jack. 1982. *More Medical Care, Better Health? An Economic Analysis of Mortality Rates.* Washington, D.C.: Urban Institute Press.

————. 1988. "Medicare Spending and Mortality Rates of the Elderly." *Inquiry* 25 (4) (winter): 485–93.

Hertz, Erica, James R. Herbert, and Joan Landon. 1994. "Social and Environmental Factors and Life Expectancy, Infant Mortality, and Maternal Mortality Rates: Results of a Cross-National Comparison." *Social Science and Medicine* 39 (1) (July): 105–14.

Lena, Hugh F., and Bruce London. 1993. "The Political and Economic Determinants of Health Outcomes: A Cross-National Analysis." *International Journal of Health Services* 23 (3): 585–602.

Lichtenberg, Frank R. 1996. "The Effect of Pharmaceutical Utilization and Innovation on Hospitalization and Mortality." NBER Working Paper 5418, January.

Moore, William J., and Robert J. Newman. 1993. "Drug Formulary Restrictions as a Cost-Containment Policy in Medicaid Programs." *Journal of Law and Economics* 36 (1–2) (April): 71–97.

Murray, Christopher J. L. 1987. "A Critical Review of International Mortality Data." *Social Science and Medicine* 25 (7): 773–81.

Nelson, Charles R., and Richard Startz. 1990. "The Distribution of the Instrumental Variables Estimator and Its *t*-Ratio When the Instrument Is a Poor One." *Journal of Business* 63 (1) (January), pt. 2: s125–40.

Newhouse, Joseph P. 1977. "Medical-Care Expenditure: A Cross-National Survey." *Journal of Human Resources* 12 (1) (winter): 115–25.

New York Times. 1991. "Gluttons for Pills. French Ask Why." January 21: A12.

Organization for Economic Cooperation and Development. OECD Health Data 96 and 98: A Comparative Analysis of 29 Countries. CD-ROM or Windows diskette.

Parkin, David, Alistair McGuire, and Brian Yule. 1987. "Aggregate Health Care Expenditures and National Income: Is Health Care a Luxury Good?" *Journal of Health Economics* 6 (2) (June): 109–27.

Peltzman, Sam. 1987. "Regulation and Health: The Case of Mandatory Prescriptions and an Extension." *Managerial and Decision Economics* 8 (1) (March): 41–46.

REFERENCES

Rodgers, G. B. 1979. "Income and Inequality as Determinants of Mortality: An International Cross-Section Analysis." *Population Studies* 33 (2): 343–51.

Shapiro, S., and M. Wilk. 1965. "An Analysis of Variance Test for Normality (Complete Samples)." *Biometrika* 52: 591–611.

Soumerai, Stephen B., Dennis Ross-Degnan, Jerry Avorn, Thomas J. McLaughlin, and Igor Choodnovskiy. 1991. "Effects of Medicaid Drug-Payment Limits on Admission to Hospitals and Nursing Homes." *New England Journal of Medicine* 325 (15) (October 10): 1072–77.

Soumerai, Stephen B., Thomas J. McLaughlin, Dennis Ross-Degnan, Christina S. Casteris, and Paola Bollini. 1994. "Effects of Limiting Medicaid Drug-Reimbursement Benefits on the Use of Psychotropic Agents and Acute Mental Health Services by Patients with Schizophrenia." *New England Journal of Medicine* 331 (10) (September 8): 650–55.

Stewart, Jr., Charles T. 1971. "Allocations of Resources to Health." *Journal of Human Resources* 6 (1) (winter): 103–22.

Szuba, Tadeusz J. 1986. "International Comparison of Drug Consumption: Impact of Prices." *Social Science and Medicine* 22 (10): 1019–25.

U.S. Congress, Office of Technology Assessment. 1993. *International Health Statistics: What the Numbers Mean for the United States—Background Paper.* OTA-BP-H-116 (November). Washington, D.C.: Government Printing Office.

Wall, Howard J. 1996. "Human Development and Income Growth in Developing Countries." *Journal of Economic Perspectives* 10 (2) (spring): 207–12.

Washington Post. 1988. "Mellowed Out in France; Tranquilizer Use Said to Be World's Highest." October 11: WH9.

Wnuk-Lipinski, Edmund, and Raymond Illsley. 1990. "International Comparative Analysis: Main Findings and Conclusions." *Social Science and Medicine* 31 (8): 879–89.

Wolfe, Barbara. 1986. "Health Status and Medical Expenditures: Is There a Link?" *Social Science and Medicine* 22 (10): 993–99.

Wolfe, Barbara, and Mary Gabay. 1987. "Health Status and Medical Expenditures: More Evidence of a Link." *Social Science and Medicine* 25 (8): 883–88.

Zweifel, Peter, and Matteo Ferrari. 1992. "Is There a Sisyphus Syndrome in Health Care?" In *Health Economics Worldwide*, edited by Peter Zweifel and H. E. Frech III. Amsterdam: Kluwer Academic Publishers, pp. 311–30.

Index

Accidents, 6

African Americans, 5

Alcohol consumption. *See also* Gender differences
  controlled, in research, 35
  data sets, 72–75, 77
  effects of, 8, 21, 36, 44, 57

Analyses. *See* Methods

Anand, Sudhir, 10–13, 15

Animal fat. *See* Diet

Auster, Richard, 4–5, 45

Australia, 30, 77. *See also* International issues

Austria, 30, 69. *See also* International issues

Babazono, Akira, 16–17, 23, 46

Baily, Martin, 13

Belgium, 30, 46, 47, 50. *See also* International issues

Bulgaria, 14. *See also* International issues

Canada, 30, 66, 69. *See also* International issues

Cancer, 13, 16, 43

Cardiovascular disease, 18

Cholelithiasis, 13

Cigarette consumption. *See also* Gender differences
  data sets, 69, 72–75, 77

effects on infant mortality, 56–57

effects on life expectancy, 44, 54, 59

effects on mortality, 7–8, 21, 33, 35, 41

measurement and control, in research, 35, 54

in richer countries, 38

Cochrane, A. L., 7–8, 44, 45, 57, 58

Convalescent homes, 17

Cultural factors, 14–15

Cutler, David, 18

Danzon, Patricia, 23, 25, 28

Data sets. *See* Methods

Degenerative diseases, 16, 43. *See also* Cancer; Heart disease

Democracy, 14–15

Denmark, 2, 23, 30. *See also* International issues

Developing countries, vii, 7, 10–12, 16, 61

Diabetes, 13

Diet. *See also* Nutrition
  animal fat in, 55, 63
  data sets, 77
  dietary guidelines, 43, 44
  dietary quality and richness, ix, 3, 15–16, 35

London, Bruce, 14–15

Males. *See* Gender differences
McClellan, Mark, 18
Medicare and Medicaid, 5, 6,
     18–19
Mental health services, 20
Methods. *See also* Elasticity
     analyses, vii–viii, 4, 47
     cross-correlations, 76
     data sets, 22, 69–77
     descriptive statistics,
          36–41
     errors and flaws, vii, 1, 9,
          11, 13–14, 15, 16–17,
          21, 61–62
     Fisher price indexes, 25,
          80 n 2
     Gini coefficient, 8
     health indicators, 28–32
     lagging, 35–36
     measurements, viii, 2–3,
          4, 23–28, 54
     research comparison,
          65–68
     sensitivity of results,
          59–60
     specification issues, 33–
          36, 80 n 2
     statistical, 4
     variables, viii
Moore, F., 7–8, 44, 45, 57, 58
Moore, William, 19
Mortality. *See also* Infant mor-
     tality
          from cardiovascular dis-
               ease, 18
          causes of, 16
          cigarette smoking and al-
               cohol consumption, 44
          cultural and political vari-
               ables, 14–15
          educational variables, 5
          environmental variables,
               5

as a health indicator, 28
income variables, 5
infectious versus degener-
     ative causes, 16
medical care variables, 5,
     7
nutrition and, 15–16
pharmaceuticals and, 12–
     13, 17–18, 21
public health and, vii, 6, 7
understatement of rates,
     6
Murder, 6
Murray, Christopher J. L., 28

National Ambulatory Medical
     Care Survey (NAMCS) Drug
     Mentions, 17–18
National Center for Health
     Statistics, 5
National Hospital Discharge
     Survey, 18
Netherlands, 31, 47, 50. *See
     also* International issues
New Hampshire, 19–20
Newhouse, Joseph, 18
New Jersey, 19
Newman, Robert, 19
New Zealand, 31, 69, 77. *See
     also* International issues
Norway, 31. *See also* Interna-
     tional issues
Nursing homes, 19
Nutrition. *See* Diet

O'Connor, Kathleen, 15–16,
     43
OECD. *See* Organization for
     Economic Cooperation and
     Development
Office of Technology Assess-
     ment (OTA), 28–29
Organization for Economic
     Cooperation and Develop-

About the Authors

H. E. FRECH III is a professor of economics at the University of California, Santa Barbara. He has been a visiting professor at the University of Chicago and at Harvard University. From 1970 to 1972, he was an economist with the U.S. Department of Health, Education, and Welfare.

Mr. Frech has published more than ninety articles and books. He is the North American editor for the *International Journal of the Economics of Business,* the series editor for "Health Economics and Public Policy" for Kluwer Academic Publishers, and a member of the editorial board of *Economic Inquiry.* He is also the author of *Competition and Monopoly in Medical Care* (AEI Press, 1996).

Mr. Frech received his doctorate in economics from the University of California, Los Angeles. He is an adjunct scholar of the American Enterprise Institute.

RICHARD MILLER is a research analyst within the Support, Planning, and Management Division of the Center for Naval Analyses in Alexandria, Virginia. He primarily focuses on studying the military health services system. Mr. Miller earned his Ph.D. in economics from the University of California at Santa Barbara in 1997. He specializes in health economics as well as in econometric analysis and labor economics.

*This book was edited by
Ann Petty of the publications staff
of the American Enterprise Institute.
The index was prepared by
Julia Petrakis.
The text was set in New Baskerville.
Coghill Composition Company
of Richmond, Virginia,
set the type,
and Edwards Brothers, Incorporated,
of Lillington, North Carolina,
printed and bound the book,
using permanent acid-free paper.*

The AEI Press is the publisher for the American Enterprise Institute for Public Policy Research, 1150 Seventeenth Street, N.W., Washington, D.C. 20036; *Christopher DeMuth,* publisher; *Ann Petty,* editor; *Leigh Tripoli,* editor; *Cheryl Weissman,* editor; *Alice Anne English,* managing editor; *Susanna Huang,* editorial production assistant.